Essentials of Pathology for Toxicologists

Paul Grasso
Former Professor of Experimental Pathology
University of Surrey
UK

with a section on Clinical Chemistry by
Sharat D. Gangolli
Visiting Professor of Toxicology
University of East London
Former Director of BIBRA Toxicology International

and a section on Haematology by
Ian Gaunt
Consultant in Toxicology

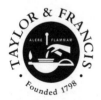

London and New York

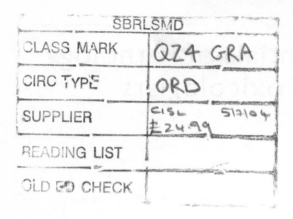
First published 2002
by Taylor & Francis
11 New Fetter Lane, London EC4P 4EE

Simultaneously published in the USA and Canada
by Taylor & Francis Inc.,
29 West 35th Street, New York, NY 10001

Taylor & Francis is an imprint of the Taylor & Francis Group

© 2002 Taylor & Francis

Typeset in Garamond by
Integra Software Services Pvt. Ltd, Pondicherry, India
Printed and bound in Great Britain by
TJ International Ltd, Padstow, Cornwall

British Library Cataloguing in Publication Data
A catalogue record for this book is available
from the British Library

Library of Congress Cataloguing in Publication Data
A catalogue record has been requested

ISBN 0–415–25980–0 (hbk)
ISBN 0–415–25795–6 (pbk)

To my wife

Contents

List of tables   ix
List of figures   xi
Acknowledgements   xiii
Preface   xv
On the threshold   xvii
Introduction   xix
The pathologist's tools   xxi
The pathologist's report   xxiii

1 Cellular pathology   **1**
    1.1   The cell and cell damage   1
    1.2   Necrosis and apoptosis   12
    1.3   Reactive responses   14

2 Tissue pathology   **17**
    2.1   Obstructive lesions   17
    2.2   Inflammation – acute   18
    2.3   Inflammation – chronic   21
    2.4   Tissue injury, restitution, repair   25

3 Cancer   **31**
    3.1   Neoplasia   31
    3.2   Causation of tumours   37

4   Immunology – an introduction   **39**
   4.1   Innate (non-specific) immunity   39
   4.2   Acquired (specific) immunity   41

5   Causation of disease   **45**
   5.1   Genetically determined   45
   5.2   Acquired – infective agents   46
   5.3   Congenital disease   47

6   Some recent advances in pathology   **49**
   6.1   Recurrent themes in pathology   50
   6.2   Apoptosis   51
   6.3   Adaptation   52
   6.4   Target organ toxicity   53
   6.5   Oncogenes   53

7   Clinical chemistry   **55**
   7.1   Enzymes   56
   7.2   Proteins in plasma   68
   7.3   Hormones and steroids in plasma   72
   7.4   Biochemical changes related to
        chemical toxicity   74
   7.5   Methodologies – general   79
   7.6   Summary and conclusion   82

8   Haematology   **87**
   8.1   Cytology   88
   8.2   Haematology and toxicology studies   89
   8.3   Historical data   93

   Glossary   99
   Further reading on pathology   155
   Further reading on clinical chemistry   159
   Further reading on haematology   161
   Index   163

Tables

1.1 Comparative composition of oedema fluid   16

2.1 Inflammatory lesion   25

3.1 Character of a tumour   33

4.1 Summary of innate and acquired immunity defenses   41

7.1 International classification of enzymes and major sub-classes   58

7.2 Intracellular location of some major enzyme systems in mammalian metabolism pathways (also included are some enzymes in the G.I. Microflora)   60

7.3 Serum enzymes of diagnostic value indicative of tissue injury   62

7.4 Enzymic processes mediating the metabolic bioactivation and detoxification of foreign compounds   64

7.5 Isoforms of the Cytochrome P-450 superfamily mediating mixed function oxidase reaction   69

7.6 Examples of proteins in plasma of potential diagnostic value for monitoring disease   70

7.7 Examples of plasma proteins as markers of tumours   72

7.8 Examples of some hypothalamic releasing hormones and their effects on anterior pituitary hormone production   73

7.9   Examples of some endocrine derived substances
       of diagnostic value   75
7.10 Changes in biochemical markers in body fluid
       indicative of target organ toxicity   80
8.1   The life cycle of red and white cells   88
8.2   Measurements commonly included in
       haematological examinations   94
8.3   Examples of measurements that may be
       included for the investigation of
       haematological effects   97

Figures

1.1 Cellular organelles – they carry out most of the
     important functions of the cell.   2
1.2 Cell nutrition.   3
1.3 Mitosis.   5
1.4 Intracellular oedema – an early marker of cell
     damage.   7
1.5 Fatty change – a marker of cell damage.   10
1.6 Programmed and random cell death.   13
2.1 A developing abscess.   19
2.2 An abscess in a portion of lung.   22
2.3 Chronic inflammation.   23
2.4 Repair by restitution.   26
2.5 Repair by fibrosis.   28
3.1 Spread of cancer in tissues (macroscopic).   32
3.2 Papilloma – a benign tumour.   33
3.3 Advanced growth by permeation of the tissue
     spaces.   34
3.4 Tumour breaching basement member prior to
     infiltration.   36
4.1 Antigen surrounded by complement and
     antibodies prior to lysis.   40
4.2 B-lymphocyte.   42
4.3 T-lymphocyte.   42
7.1 Bioactivation and detoxification scheme for
     foreign chemicals.   66

Acknowledgements

The authors would like to extend their thanks to their friends and colleagues for their help and encouragement in preparing the text; to Carole Grasso for contributing the section on immunology; to Suzanne Grasso and Joe Lee-Brown for their excellent artwork and to Maria Grasso for her invaluable advice on the book cover.

In addition, the authors would like to pay an especial thank you to IUPAC for allowing the reproduction of part of their Glossary that was relevant to this book.

Preface

This book is based on a series of lectures on pathology given to students of the MSc (Tox) at one of the South East's universities. This course was the first post-graduate course in Toxicology in Europe and a selected group of scientists from a wide group of disciplines was given the task of drawing up a curriculum for the course. Because toxicology is a multidisciplinary subject, the topics in the curriculum were selected to reflect this diversity. Likewise, students admitted to the course had the most varied scientific background – analytical chemists, biochemists, physiologists, medics and vets and the occasional nuclear physicist.

From the start, pathology presented greater teaching difficulties than any other subject. Complaints were made that pathology as taught in the course was virtually incomprehensible. These complaints came principally from students with little or no background in any of the biological sciences. Surprisingly, complaints were also received from students equipped to follow the subject. These complaints chiefly concerned the short time allocated to the subject. Unfortunately, time is restricted in the course because of the wide range of subjects that have to be covered to satisfy the curriculum.

Students sought refuge in books of pathology then available to complement their lectures and found to their disappointment that these were of little assistance – they were written for medics and vets and the pathological detail was far above that required for the toxicology students. Since that time, a few books have appeared on pathology aimed at the toxicologist and are of some assistance for those without background in biology. These publications are mainly concerned with descriptions of pathological changes by some specific test substance. They assume that the reader is already familiar with the principles of pathology so that the tyros are not really better off, particularly, if they have had no pathological background.

Based on experience gained over the years, we have ventured to put together a handbook which we hope will be of assistance to the aspiring student in grasping the fundamental principles of pathology and learn how to apply them as the situation requires.

In the preparation of this book, particular attention has been given to general pathology but selected examples from systemic pathology are included to show that pathology is not an isolated entity but serves as the foundation for understanding the nature of the lesion they come across. The time constraint meant that the lectures had to be kept very short and the material strictly relevant. In compiling the book these properties were kept in mind.

As the work progressed, we realised the need for having two more subjects – Clinical Chemistry and Haematology.

Clinical chemistry has been introduced to remind the young student that the morphologic pictures seen by the microscope have their origins at molecular level.

Books on haematology for toxicologists are very rare indeed; our contribution will help to fill the gap.

Paul Grasso
Sharat D. Gangolli
Ian Gaunt

On the threshold

For the average student, crossing the threshold of a pathology laboratory must be quite an experience if not a cultural shock. They would search in vain for any imposing pieces of laboratory hardware that fill the rooms of most modern laboratories. Instead, they would see a few pieces of equipment designed for the sole purpose of "fixing" tissue in formalin and then embedding it in wax. Further enquires would reveal that the waxed tissue is sliced into thin sections ($5\,\mu$) and mounted on a glass slide for examination by the pathologist. At this stage, the section is transparent and colourless so that the internal structure of the cells cannot be identified by light or electron-microscopy. To overcome this difficulty, the sections are stained. A variety of colourings are used for this purpose, the most popular being haematoxilin and eosin (HE). The tyro cannot help noticing rows of coloured bottles on the shelves – neither fail to notice the coloured blotches on the benches... some disaster to user – some unlucky tyro?

Introduction

Pathology is usually defined as the science of disease. Disease is a disturbance of normal bodily function beyond the ability of the organism to cope. In other words, the organism has lost it's ability to adapt to specific changes. The dictionary defines adaptation as "to modify, to make fit or suitable". In life, there is a need for constant change in organ function to keep up with a constantly changing environment. The extent to which these changes occur depends on the nature and severity of the environmental change and the ability of the organism to cope with it. The response is dependent largely on the functional reserve. Excessive demands on this reserve herald the onset of pathology. How does the mammalian organism adapt? The result is in the realm of physiology, a science committed among other objectives to define the boundary between the normal and abnormal and we could venture to put forward a "rule of thumb" to answer that question:

1   An increase in enzyme activity. This occurs spectacularly in the liver of the rat and mouse but occurs also in other species including man.
2   Increase in the number of functional cells – organ enlarges.
3   Increase in the size of the cells – cell enlarges (e.g. hypertrophy of cardiac muscle in athletes or in hypertensives).

4 Recruitment – In the resting state most cells or functional units are at a low ebb of activity. In an emergency, these are called upon to increase activity thus enhancing the functional capacity of the organ (e.g. CNS).

The four points mentioned above are not exclusive to any specific tissue or anatomical site. They apply equally well to protein synthesis, hormonal stimulation and receptor mechanisms.

Pathology has been likened to a bridge between the basic sciences and clinical and veterinary medicine. Indeed, over the years, we have seen a plethora of special investigations aimed at providing additional information to clarify specific diagnostic problems in medical or veterinary practice. This allows a more accurate treatment to be made. For example, a patient with chest pain is first seen by a clinician who may require further information on the patient's condition by the use of enzymes, electronics and/or X-rays (see Chapter 7). In another example, a patient presents with a swelling of the neck. After clinical examination a biopsy is taken. The pathologist sees a section of it and conveys the result to the clinician. Further examination may be carried out – chemistry, bacteriology etc., they help in forming a definitive diagnosis. The so-called ancillary investigations (see Chapter 7) constitute the application of basic science to pathology.

The pathologist's tools

At the end of examination of the tissues, the pathologist is requested to present a report. To enable the pathologist to perform this task, a set of "tools" is required consisting of:

1 a good clinical report;
2 relevant laboratory investigations;
3 biopsy/necropsy report;
4 histology;
5 electron microscopy; and
6 biochemistry/molecular biology.

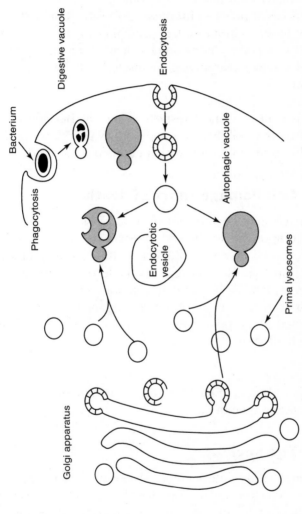

Bacterium

Digestive vacuole

Phagocytosis

Endocytosis

Autophagic vacuole

Endocytotic vesicle

Prima lysosomes

Golgi apparatus

Redrawn: Bruce, A., Dennis, B., Julian Martin, R., Robins, K., James, W. (eds). The Molecular Biology of the Cell. Garland Publishing, New York and London (1983).

Figure 1.2 Cell nutrition.

Mitosis is divided into a number of stages (Figure 1.3):

1 Resting stage;
2 Early prophase – centriole divided and nuclear DNA rearranging itself into chromosomes;
3 Centrioles at poles – chromosomes visibly doubled;
4 Metaphase – chromosomes arranging themselves at the equator of cell – chromosomes clearly identifiable; and
5 Chromosomes rearranging themselves into two daughter nuclei.

Meiosis is similar in most respect to mitosis but consists of two consecutive cell divisions without DNA synthesis period. This is the form of division which germ cells undergo.

1.1.2 Cell damage short of death

Cell damage may be inflicted on one or other of the sub-cellular components of the cell by toxic chemicals. Some of these exert their detrimental effect on the cell by interfering with the function of a specific organelle (e.g. fluoroacetate interferes with mitochondrial respiration) others like nitrogen mustard react with all of the cell organelles.

For practical purposes, we can divide cell damage into that which affects:

- the nucleus;
- the cytoplasmic organelles and the cytoplasm; and
- the plasma membrane.

1.1.3 The nucleus

No morphological changes in the nucleus have been described by light or electron microscopy following sublethal damage by external agents. Investigations by specialised techniques for example, by tests for DNA repair, mutagenic changes *in vitro* or *in vivo*, and some of the more recently introduced

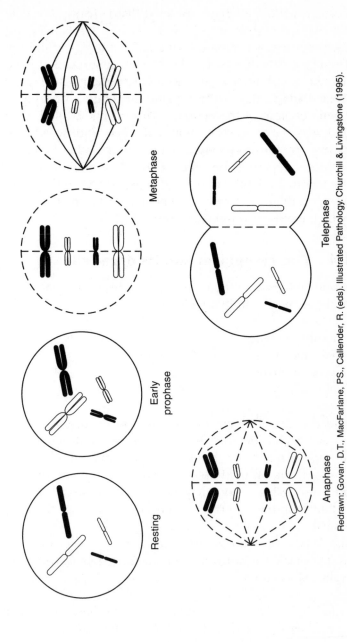

Resting

Early
prophase

Metaphase

Anaphase

Telephase

Redrawn: Govan, D.T., MacFarlane, PS., Callender, R. (eds). Illustrated Pathology. Churchill & Livingstone (1995).

Figure 1.3 Mitosis.

molecular techniques have revealed that considerable damage may occur and that the nucleus has a relatively vast capacity for repair compared with that of the rest of the cell.

The chemicals that induce DNA damage are called genotoxic. One consequence of genotoxicity is the possibility that nuclear damage may be misrepaired leading to a change in the gene content of the genome. This change (called mutagenic) may have a very short existence and so of very limited scope for producing damage. On the other hand, the misrepaired gene may become incorporated with the normal genes where it might multiply and cause cancer. If the misrepair occurs in gonadal tissues, genetic defects may occur and may be passed on to the offspring.

1.1.4 The cytoplasm and its organelles

The principal types of injury that occurs from the administration of chemicals can be divided into:

1 cloudy swelling;
2 hydropic change;
3 vacuolar change; and
4 fatty change.

Before the development of the electron microscope (EM), there was a considerable debate whether changes occurred at all. It is now known from EM studies that cloudy swelling is a form of mild to moderate intracellular oedema (Figure 1.4). This lesion may be reversible or progressive depending on the severity of damaged or dose of the toxic chemical.

The types of damage mentioned above can be seen morphologically in conventionally stained paraffin sections by light microscopy.

1 *Cloudy swelling* is the term used to describe a cell which is enlarged, pale and has a fine granular cyto-

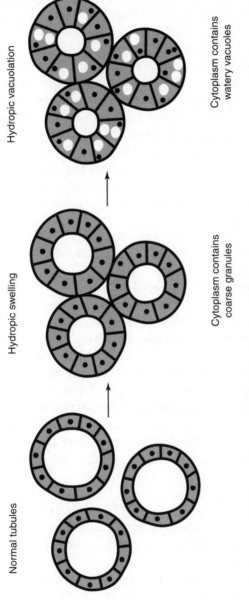

Normal tubules

Hydropic swelling

Cytoplasm contains
coarse granules

Hydropic vacuolation

Cytoplasm contains
watery vacuoles

Figure 1.4 Intracellular oedema – an early marker of cell damage.

plasm. The nuclear structure and size are preserved ultrastructurally. Cloudy swelling has been associated with mitochondrial swelling or with dilatation of the endoplasmic reticulum.

2 *Vacuolar change* consists of multiple, fluid filled, roughly spherical vacuoles in the cytoplasm. Nuclear structure normal; ultrastructurally there is a localised loss of cytoplasm – the vacuoles are not surrounded by a definable membrane but by ragged cytoplasm.

3 *Hydropic change* is the term reserved for the most severe form of intracellular oedema. The cell is usually dilated grossly with formation of large vacuoles that are irregular in size, and are surrounded by a rough, ragged border of shrunken cytoplasm. The nucleus shows clear evidence of shrinking and condensation (pyknosis). The large and irregular vacuoles of hydropic change contain cytoplasm fragments and have no clear edge.

4 *Fatty change* denotes neutral fat occurring in small amounts in the healthy mammalian liver and kidney and represents fat in transit from sites of absorption and synthesis to sites of storage or utilisation for the provision of energy. This fat is demonstrable by appropriate histochemical stains. An excess of fat is sometimes seen after the administration of toxic chemicals, particularly in liver and kidney. This may mean either that the metabolism of the cell is deranged so that it cannot utilise the fat for energy or process it for export. In both instances, the fat accumulation denotes a pathological effect.

Excess triglyceride may appear in the liver of rats if they are given an excess of fat in the diet or else a fat that either cannot be fully broken down (e.g. brominated oils) or else broken slowly (e.g. eurcic acid). This is really a sort of "storage" phenomenon. It is arguable whether this sort of change denotes a pathological change – toxicologically it is undesirable.

As shown in Figure 1.5, fat accumulation change may result from a defective oxygen supply to a particular tissue. This phenomenon is best observed in the human heart muscle exposed to chronic anaemia.

1.1.5 Some slowly progressive tissue damage

1 Melanin occurs naturally in melanocytes, brain cells and in basal layer of the skin in pigmented and white races. In most other situations, it is a sign of pathological change.

2 Lipofuscin is generally known as "wear and tear" pigment and in man, it occurs typically in brown atrophy of the heart. (This condition is found in man in severe starvation and in chronic wasting diseases such as pulmonary tuberculosis, cancer and chronic septic states.) It is now known that lipofuscin results from the polymerisation of lipidperoxides and is indicative of some abnormality of lipid metabolism. It is uncertain how lipofuscin acquires its yellow coloration.

   Lipofuscinosis occurs in most tissues in rats maintained on a Vitamin E deficient diet for most of their lifetime. It has also been found in the liver of rats fed agents which induce peroxisomal proliferation.

   Lipofuscin contains no Fe but has strong reducing properties. These help to distinguish lipofuscin from haemosiderin which is rich in Fe and has no reducing properties.

3 Haemosiderin is a golden yellow pigment and is derived from haemoglobin. It is present within macrophages at the site of an old haemorrhage. In pathological conditions involving lysis of erythrocytes, a marked increase occurs in spleen, liver and bone-marrow.

4 Bile-pigments feature infrequently in toxicological studies in rodents. They may appear in liver if there is

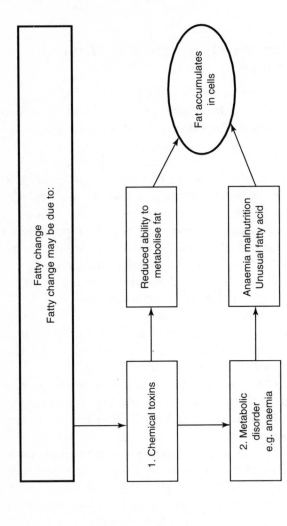

Figure 1.5 Fatty change – a marker of cell damage.

Fatty change
Fatty change may be due to:

1. Chemical toxins → Reduced ability to metabolise fat

2. Metabolic disorder e.g. anaemia → Anaemia malnutrition Unusual fatty acid

Fat accumulates in cells

obstruction to the bile duct or if they cannot be removed from the liver due to some enzymatic defect associated with their transportation and excretion.

5 Calcification: Calcium has an affinity for damaged and dying cells. In most instances, deposits occur in single cells but if cell damage involves several contiguous cells a large calcium deposit forms at the site (e.g. atheromatous lesions). This type of calcification is called dystrophic calcification.

Calcium may be deposited in tissues as a result of high serum calcium (e.g. hypervitaminosis D or hyperparathyroidism). This type of calcification is known as metastatic calcification.

1.1.6 Storage disorders

"Storage disorders" have been identified and shown to be due to some enzyme deficiency. They are usually congenital. The material "stored" is usually the same as that forming the tissues. There are no toxicity reports of chemicals producing this condition.

1.1.7 Some other changes indicative of cell damage

1.1.7.1 Hyalyne

Hyalyne refers to a microscopic appearance of an abnormally homogenous area which usually stains bright red with eosin. It may occur intra- or extra-cellularly. The term describes the appearance of tissue stained with haematoxilin but does not specify its nature. (e.g. the $\alpha\,2\mu$ protein in unleaded gasoline).

1.1.7.2 Fibrinoid change

In some pathological conditions, generally of an autoimmune character, tissue stains more intensely than expected and their texture resembles that of fibrin. This abnormality is usually seen in the walls of blood vessels or in collagenous connective tissue, sometimes accompanied by an inflammatory reaction. Fibrinoid change may be due to fibrin or it may be due to immune complexes deposited on the walls of the blood vessels.

1.1.7.3 Amyloid

Basically it is a paraprotein which is deposited extracellularly on the reticulin network of organs. Its progressive accumulation "chokes" off the surrounding parenchymal cells. It forms in chronic debilitating disease e.g. Hodgkin's disease, tuberculosis.

1.2 NECROSIS AND APOPTOSIS

Necrosis is usually defined as the death of a cell or cells in continuity with living tissue. Cell death results from an interruption of one or more of the processes which maintain its life (Figure 1.6). The commonest causes are:

1   deprivation of blood supply;
2   compression;
3   physical agents (e.g. radiation, solid objects etc.);
4   infection; and
5   chemicals.

Macroscopically dead tissue may remain firm in consistency (coagulative necrosis) or it may liquefy (colliquative necrosis e.g. an abscess or damaged brain). If necrosis involves a large mass of tissue, it is called gangrene. This mass of dead tissue may undergo putrefaction by bacterial (saprophytic) invasion. This is called "wet" gangrene. "Dry" gangrene is said to occur when the dead tissue shrivels and

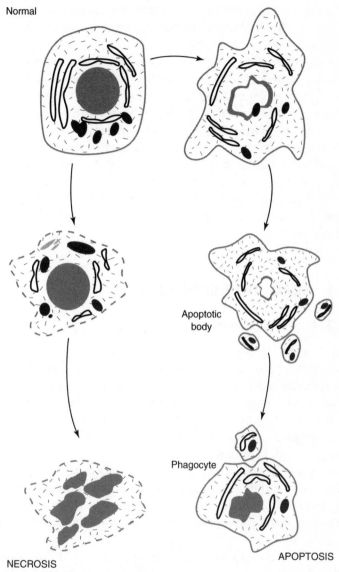

Normal

Apoptotic
body

Phagocyte

NECROSIS

APOPTOSIS

Redrawn: Kumar, V., Cottram, R., Robinson, S. (eds). Basic Pathology. W.P. Saunders,
New York and London (1997).

Figure 1.6 Programmed and random cell death.

shrinks, becomes black and dry like the skin of an Egyptian mummy. It also occurs when there is a blockage of a large artery in the limbs. No bacterial infection occurs in "dry" gangrene.

Apoptosis: Since the late 1980s, the term apoptosis has been accepted in pathology to mean programmed cell death. As a result of intense studies, it is now generally agreed that apoptosis affects single cells, whereas necrosis affects groups of cells. Necrosis elicits an inflammatory response while apoptosis does not do so. The nucleus becomes denser in apoptosis whereas it undergoes lysis or karyorhexis in necrosis. Apoptosis is regarded as physiological – the cell dies according to a scheduled programme whereas necrosis is a random event. There are no visible macroscopic changes in apoptosis.

1.3   REACTIVE RESPONSES

1.3.4   Hypertrophy

An increase in size of an organ is classed as hypertrophy. The term is also applied to individual cells. Enlarged organs are heavier than their normal counterpart and it is now customary to weigh enlarged organs. It must be remembered however, that organ enlargement may be due to some pathological process. Thus, in brain oedema the organ becomes heavier than normal.

In some circumstances, it may be necessary to produce objective evidence of cell enlargement. Histologically, this is difficult to undertake but acceptable evidence may be obtained by counting the cells in sections in corresponding areas in test and controls.

The term hypertrophy is being applied to EM if an organelle is present in greater amounts than in controls. Thus, phenobarbitone induces a striking increase in ER which has been classed as hypertrophic.

1.3.2   Hyperplasia

It is an increase in a number of cells in an organ or tissue. It is often associated with organ enlargement so that an increase in size of an organ may be due to an increase in the number or size of its constituent cells, or of both simultaneously.

Hyperplasia could be either (a) restorative; or (b) physiologic. Restorative hyperplasia occurs after a massive loss of the constituent cells in an organ as a result of an operation, treatment, or trauma. Whereas, physiologic hyperplasia occurs in organs that are the target for hormonal activity or that participate whenever there is an increased metabolic demand.

1.3.3   Metaplasia

Means the transformation of one type of epithelium to another. For example, the trachea and large bronchi in smokers lose their goblet and ciliated cells as well as mucus and become lined by stratified squamous epithelium. The reason for this change is not clear but its association with chronic irritation suggests that it represents a change of a delicate epithelium to a more robust one.

Metaplasia may occur in the other direction. The lower end of the oesophagus may lose its stratified squamous epithelium and be replaced by intestinal type epithelium. Metaplasia is not always beneficial, for example; the protection of the mucus carpet is lost in the transition from respiratory to squamous epithilium.

1.3.4   Atrophy

Means cell shrinkage. This may occur from compression and poor blood supply. The lesion is reversible.

1.3.5   Oedema

Oedema is the name given to an excess of the fluid which surrounds each cell. This fluid is called extracellular fluid

(ECF). Under physiological conditions its main function is to bring in nutrients and take away products of xenobiotic and intermediary metabolism. In this state, it is called a transudate. Under pathological conditions more extracellular fluid than normal is formed which can be only accommodated by an expansion of the local ECF. Protein and cells find their way into the ECF from blood capillaries increasing the demand for space. In this condition, it is called an exudate (Table 1.1).

Table 1.1 Comparative composition of oedema fluid

Item	Transudate	Exudate
Protein type	Low – less than (30 g/l) Low molecular weight	High – more than (30 g/l) High molecular weight similar to that found in plasma
	Only albumen	
Fibrinogen	Absent	Present – may clot
Lactate dehydrogenase (LDH)	Less than 200 iu	More than 200 iu
Cells	Absent	Present

Chapter 2

Tissue pathology

2.1 OBSTRUCTIVE LESIONS

2.1.1 Thrombosis

Blood may coagulate (clots) both internally (in blood vessels) and externally. Outside the body, its principal function is to staunch blood loss. When blood clots internally, it may produce an obstruction and the parent organism can be, and generally is, in a very poor state of health (heart infarct).

A mass of coagulated blood outside the body is called a clot, when it occurs inside the body it is called a thrombus. This distinction is not always kept in practice. Thrombi are formed by the deposition of blood clotting factors (platelets, fibrin) on to a rough surface of a blood vessel. This leads to the gradual build-up of fibrin which may end-up as thrombi locking end-arteries.

An end-artery is a blood vessel of medium size between a branch of the aorta and a small artery – e.g. arteriole. It is so called because it has no collateral vessels through which any trapped blood may escape (as e.g. skeletal muscle).

Blocking of the blood flow means that the tissue supplied by the blocked artery is deprived of its blood supply and quickly (or sometimes slowly) dies. This type of death is called an infarction.

In internal organs, the infarct appears as a dark grey tissue surrounded by an even darker ring of tissue. This ring of tissue is histologically seen to be an inflammatory reaction. The rest of the tissue stains very lightly with eosin but preserves the original structure – the infarct appears as "a shadow of its former self".

If the infarct occurs on the body surface, it may get infected and becomes known as "wet" gangrene (massive tissue death with bacterial infection). If the infarct is not infected then the gangrene is called "dry" gangrene (mummyfication).

2.1.2 More on infarction

Infarction occurs wherever there is a disruption of the blood flow. Infarcts may be red or white. In red infarcts, the affected area is full of blood, hence the red colour. Red infarct occurs when the blood supply is interrupted by a vein or veins. In a white infarct, the blood entrapped in the affected area gradually loses the blood supply originally there. A white infarct is normally shrunken.

At necropsy, the infarct is usually wedge shaped with the apex pointing inwards.

2.1.3 Embolism

As mentioned in Section 2.1.1, blood may coagulate if it comes into contact with a rough endothelial surface of blood vessels. The clot thus formed may remain static or parts of it may detach themselves and lodge in distant regions of the blood vascular systems. These fragments are called emboli.

2.2 INFLAMMATION – ACUTE

Inflammation is arguably the most important defence system developed in the mammalian organism. It acts as an efficient protective shield for warding off any agent likely to inflict damage to the host.

This process has been the subject of intense study from the time of Celsius (30 B.C.). Its popularity is probably due to its dramatic onset in an organ which is readily accessible for examination.

To begin with let us consider the skin at or shortly after a damaging agent has established itself and let us call it the epicentre (Figure 2.1). This epicentre, usually not bigger

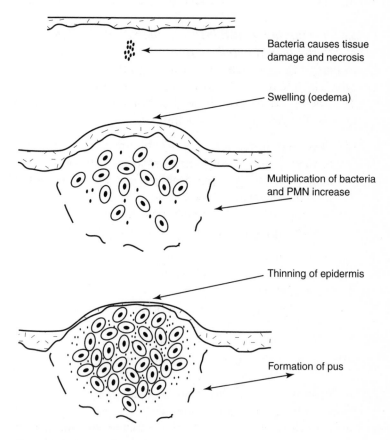

Bacteria causes tissue damage and necrosis

Swelling (oedema)

Multiplication of bacteria and PMN increase

Thinning of epidermis

Formation of pus

Figure 2.1 A developing abscess.

than a pin's head, is covered with fibrin and appears dark. It will soon be surrounded by a ring of redness which is swollen, tender and warmer to the touch than surrounding skin. Throbbing may also be an early feature. A few hours later, the ring of redness is replaced by a ring of blueness (cyanosis) but the swelling and heat remain. The ring of redness now surrounds the damaged tissue. If the invasive agent is virulent then the tissue at the epicentre become necrotic and the surrounding concentric rings become much more marked. At the periphery of the ring of redness, the tissue is normal.

The changes mentioned above have a histological basis:

1   *Redness throbbing and heat (an increased blood flow due to arteriolar and capillary dilatation)* – hyperaemia due in part to the increased blood flow to the area.
2   *Swelling* – excessive formation of interstitial fluid (IF). The increased formation of this fluid is due to several factors, the principal ones being:

   (a) increased formation due to an imbalance between formation and absorption (formation > absorption);
   (b) increased capillary permeability leading to increased protein – formation of exudate; and
   (c) free passage of blood cells pass into interstitial fluid, (polymorphs, monocytes and/or lymphocytes).

3   *Cyanosis (blueness)* – loss of oxygenated red blood cells due to stagnation of capillary flow, caused by capillary dilatation and damage.
4   *Pain* – oedema compressing peripheral nerves.
5   *Loss of function* – to ease pain.

The end point of the inflammatory process may be:

1   an abscess (an accumulation of dead polymorphs surrounded by granulation tissue);
2   an ulcer (loss of epithelium and formation of granulation tissue);

3   resolution (return of tissue to normal);
4   fibrosis (replacement of tissue destroyed in the inflammatory process by connective tissue also known as scar tissue); and
5   systemic invasion may occur if the invading organism is virulent or the host is debilitated. Usually a fatal complication.

Some additional points:

1   The inflammatory process is the same irrespective of the tissue where it is taking place.
2   The site of the inflammatory process may determine which component dominates, for example – oedema is very prominent in inflammatory lung disease because of the spongy character of the host tissue (Figure 2.2). Oedema is virtually absent in bone infections because the small space between the periosteum and bone. Pain is, on the other hand, a very prominent feature of bone infection. Some special types of inflammation are:

   (a) *Suppurative* (*exudate rich in pus*) – seen in lesions by pyogenic organisms.
   (b) *Catarrh* (*inflammation of the mucous membrane*) – oedema prominent.
   (c) *Exudative* – marked by the excessive formation of fibrin and by intercellular fluid containing blood protein and blood cells.
   (d) *Haemorrhagic* – exudate tinged with blood.

2.3 INFLAMMATION – CHRONIC

In the previous chapter we saw that one of the end-points of acute inflammation was chronic inflammation (Figure 2.3). The term chronic is used by clinicians to denote that the affliction of the patient is likely to have a prolonged course

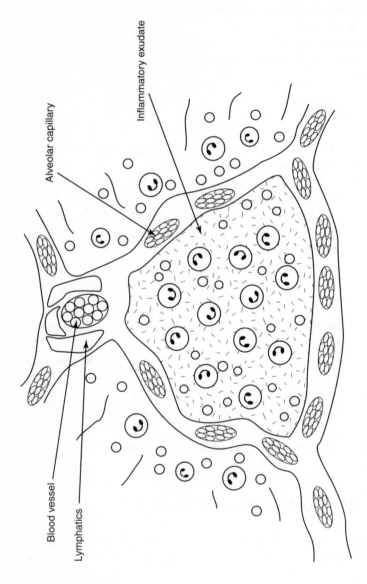

Inflammatory exudate

Alveolar capillary

Blood vessel

Lymphatics

Figure 2.2 An abscess in a portion of lung.

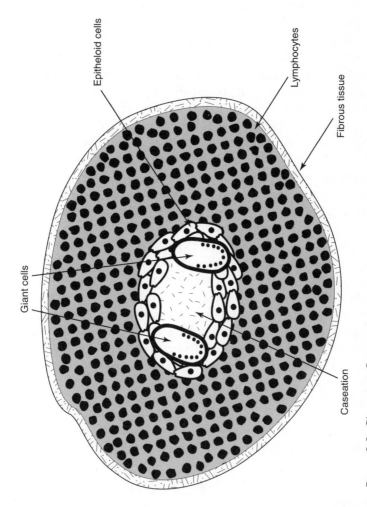

Epitheloid cells

Lymphocytes

Fibrous tissue

Giant cells

Caseation

Figure 2.3 Chronic inflammation.

as opposed to the acute disease, which runs a much shorter course. The macroscopic characteristics recall those of acute inflammation but are much milder. Microscopically the picture is very different from that of acute inflammation. Whereas the polymorph is the predominant cell in acute inflammation, the macrophage and fibroblast are the predominant cells in chronic inflammation. Capillary formation (granulation tissue) is a predominant feature of the later stages of acute inflammation. It is much less evident in chronic inflammation.

In fact, the principal characteristic of chronic inflammation is the local infiltration with macrophages and fibroblasts and other cell types with strong histogenetic links with them – the epithelioid cell and the histiocyte. The epithelioid cell is so called because its flattened appearance recalls the squamous (flat) cells of many epithelia (e.g. skin). The histiocyte resembles closely the macrophage but contains no ingested material. It is thought that both the histiocyte and epithelioid cells are important in immune reactions designed to limit or eliminate the causative agent. Their precise function is at the moment unclear but there is evidence that their role involves the "processing and presentation" of antigens to lymphocytes. There is another type of cell, which is unmistakable – foreign body giant cell. These cells come about by the fusion of macrophages and are meant to ingest particulate matter which otherwise would elude the hosts defences.

The chronic inflammatory lesion is referred to as a granuloma (Table 2.1). It consists basically of a local and variable accumulation of macrophages, histiocytes, epithelioid cells and fibroblasts proliferating together with variable amounts of plasma cells and lymphocytes. The variability of these is very great indeed so that the histological picture can vary enormously from one causative agent to another.

In toxicology, the commonest causes of granulomas are the mineral dusts e.g. talc, asbestos, silica. If inhaled by experimental animals, granulomas develop in the lung. If

Table 2.1 Inflammatory lesion

	Acute	Chronic
Cytology	Polymorphs	Macrophages and fibroblasts
Duration	A few weeks/days	Months/years
Granulation tissue	Prominent	Inconspicuous
Capillary formation	Prominent	Inconspicuous
Granulomas	Absent	Prominent

injected parenterally, the granuloma develops at the site of injection of the dust.

2.4 TISSUE INJURY, RESTITUTION, REPAIR

Tissue damage may be caused by a variety of agents, some of which are mentioned in Section 5.2. Tissue damage usually, but not invariably, results in tissue death. In the normal healthy state, the demise of the cells is followed by an attempt at replacement. The process of replacement of tissue of the same kind is known as restitution and that of replacement by scar tissue is known as repair (Figure 2.4).

2.4.1 Restitution

Let us take as an example, an incised wound of the skin. Incised wounds usually result from a sharp instrument, such as a knife, and are moderately deep.

The first effect after incision is severe bleeding due to the severance of the blood vessels in the area. The wound becomes filled with blood which eventually (in about 10 min) coagulates due to the deposition of fibrin. Fibrin

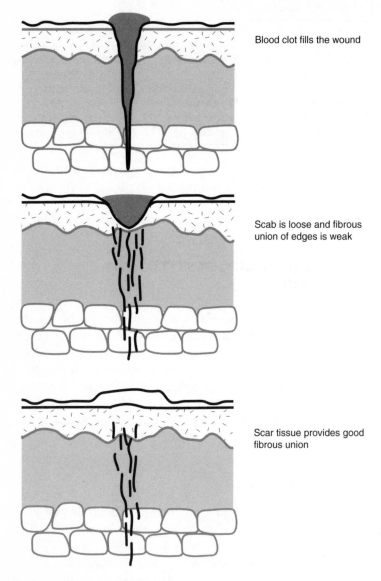

Blood clot fills the wound

Scab is loose and fibrous union of edges is weak

Scar tissue provides good fibrous union

Figure 2.4 Repair by restitution.

is a fibrous protein and serves as a scaffolding for restitution to take place. The first event in this line is the appearance of inflammatory cells (polymorphs, macrophages, lymphocytes). These cells gradually remove the fibrin plug so as to allow fibroblasts to come into the area and begin the process of restitution. This process takes place throughout the entire depth of the wound simultaneously (Figure 2.5).

After a few days, the site of damage consists of fibroblast and collagen and is difficult to distinguish from normal surrounding cells with one exception – the covering epidermis is usually thinner than the surrounding integument and has no appendages (hair follicles, sebaceous glands).

A small amount of damage in internal organs is repaired in the same way – i.e. the damaged cells are removed and replaced by cells of the same type and appearance. These changes restore the appearance of the damaged part so that they cannot be distinguished readily from surrounding tissue.

2.4.2 Repair

When the loss of tissue is extensive the process discussed in Section 2.4.1 is considerably modified but the basic principle is the same – restoring the continuity of the tissue.

If bleeding is severe then priority has to be given to stop the haemorrhage. The fibrin clot that has formed at the site of damage is gradually removed and is replaced by granulation tissue.

Repair begins at the bottom of the wound where the walls are in close proximity to each other so that the distance between the cells (chiefly the fibroblasts) can be easily bridged. The process then moves upwards as the fibroblasts contract and gradually seal the wound. The process is like the action of a zip fastener. As the healing process comes close to the surface, it is covered by skin epithelium. This covering appears to be important since the healing process

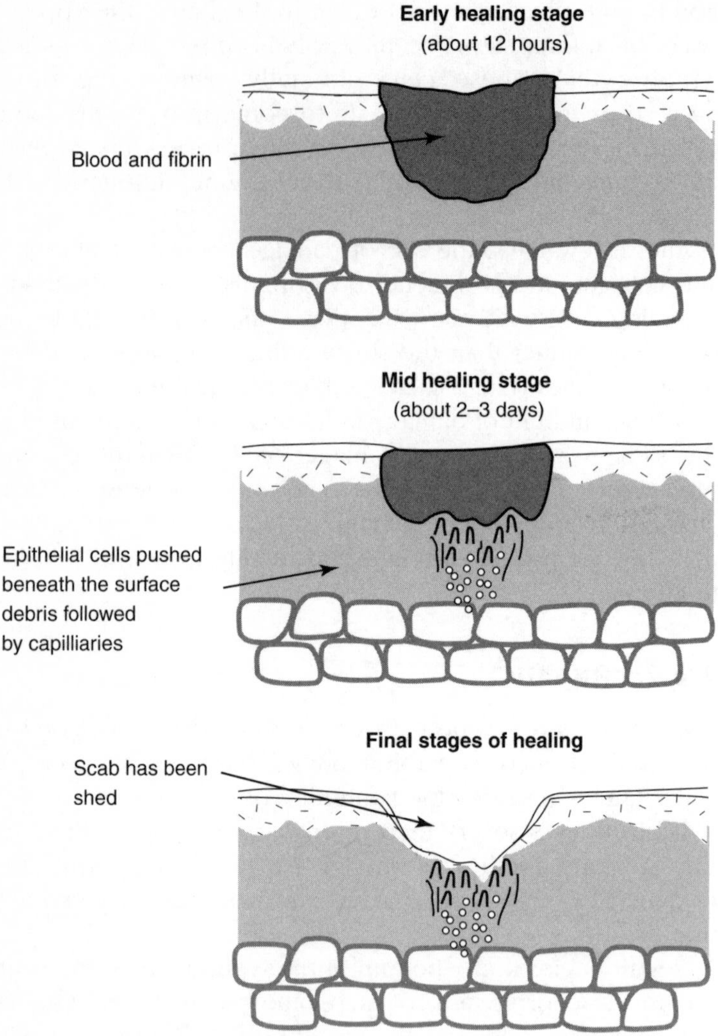

Early healing stage
(about 12 hours)

Blood and fibrin

Mid healing stage
(about 2–3 days)

Epithelial cells pushed
beneath the surface
debris followed
by capilliaries

Final stages of healing

Scab has been
shed

Figure 2.5 Repair by fibrosis.

cannot take place adequately if the epithelial covering is damaged.

The process called "restoring", restores tissues to their pristine condition – not so the process called repair. In this process, the loss of tissue is made up by granulation tissue and leaves a scar tissue behind.

Chapter 3

Cancer

3.1 NEOPLASIA

Neoplasia is a disorder of cell growth. This growth occurs by cell division and in this respect neoplastic growth resembles that of hyperplasia. In hyperplasia, cell division is strictly controlled whereas in neoplasia it is uncontrolled (Figure 3.1).

The classical definition of neoplasia is that of Rupert Willis who wrote that "a neoplasm is an abnormal mass of tissue the growth of which exceeds and is uncoordinate with that of normal tissue and persists in the same excessive manner after cessation of the stimuli which brought it about".

A shorter definition of a neoplasm is a growth which is persistent, progressive, and purposeless.

Tumours can be classified either by their biological behaviour or by their taxonomic appearance.

Biological behaviour:

- rate of growth;
- invasion – infiltration into neighbouring organs – may eventually replace them; and
- metastasis – tumour cells detach themselves from the parent growth and settle in a distant organ.

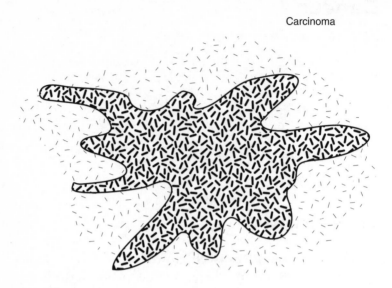

Figure 3.1 Spread of cancer in tissues (macroscopic).

3.1.1   Taxonomy

- cell type;
- site of origin; and
- architectural characteristics.

In the case of malignant tumours, one needs to know how far it has spread (*the stage*) and how poorly differentiated it is (*the grade*). The main features of benign and malignant tumours are briefly set out in Table 3.1.

The typical macroscopic appearance of a benign tumour reflects its slow growth. It tends to be round, well demarcated from surrounding tissues and sometimes clearly encapsulated. Necrosis is uncommon but can occur especially if blood vessels are compressed (Figure 3.2).

Table 3.1 Character of a tumour

Malignant	Benign	Notes
Invades local tissue and goes into lymphatics and blood vessels	Remains *in situ*	Malignant tumours spread – their most important property
Rate of growth	Grows slowly	Grows fast
Capsule	Usually complete and easy to identify	Rarely present – when present, it is irregular
Effects on adjacent tissue	Compression of vessels and nerves	Destruction of normal tissue

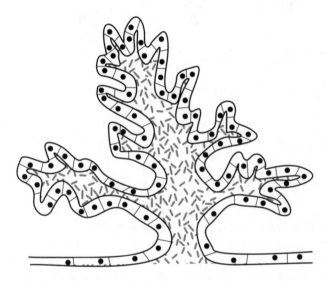

Figure 3.2 Papilloma – a benign tumour.

Malignant tumours tend to be poorly demarcated with irregular margins. The presence of a capsule is rare. Necrosis is commonly seen in malignant tumours. Metastases frequently occur in malignant tumours (Figure 3.3). This brief outline

Malignant cells permeating spaces

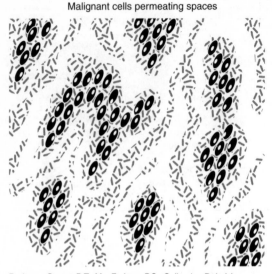

Redrawn: Govan, D.T., MacFarlane, P.S., Callender, R. (eds).
Illustrated Pathology. Churchill & Livingstone (1995).

Figure 3.3 Advanced growth by permeation of the tissue spaces.

shows how much can be learnt by the hand lens. Still more
can be learnt by the addition of light microscopy findings.

3.1.2   Histological characteristics

The architecture of a benign tumour tends to be similar to
that of the parent tissue and the cells closely resemble the
parent cells forming glands or ducts, or keratin, or connective tissue elements, (e.g. muscle or bone) depending on
their cell of origin: invasion is absent. In benign tumours, the
cells are well-differentiated have a normal nuclear cytoplasmic ratio and a smooth outline. The nuclei have a normal
complement of chromosomes (i.e. they are euploid).

   In malignant tumours, differentiation is variable so that
architectural relationships with the tissue of origin may be
difficult to recognise. Some tumours lack all features of

differentiation and these are described as anaplastic tumours. Mitoses are usually present and may be abnormal. These processes are heralded by a breakage of the basement membrane (Figure 3.4). The nuclei tend to be large and there is an increase in the nuclear/cytoplasmic ratio i.e. there seems to be more nucleus in relation to the amount of cytoplasm present. The nuclei tend to stain more heavily – a situation called hyperchromasia. In chromosome studies, malignant tumours often show population of cells with an abnormal number of chromosomes (aneuploidy).

3.1.3 More on taxonomy

The epithelial tumours are called papillomas if they are benign and carcinomas if they are malignant. Tumours which arise from secretory or ductal epithelium are called adenocarcinomas.

The term polyp is applied to a mass of tissue which arises from an epithelial surface and may be either benign, malignant or in some instances, of a chronic inflammatory nature (e.g. nasal polyp). A papilloma possesses frond-like outgrowths arising from the epithelial surface and is usually benign.

An annular tumour is one which encircles the lumen of a hollow organ and sometimes seen in some types of intestinal neoplasia – this type of tumour is locally invasive. If the tumour is soft, it is called enchephaloid; if it is hard, it is called scirrhous. Scirrhous tumours contain a very high content of fibrous tissue. The fibrous tissue is not malignant in itself but a reaction to the tumour.

Tumours of the skin are called squamous cell carcinomas, because the cell type is flat and resembles a squame (a scale). Tumours of the bladder are called transitional cell carcinomas – they appear morphologically to lie between the skin cells and the glandular ones. Tumours of the connective tissue are called sarcomas. If they arise from the areolar tissue they are called fibrosarcoma, if they arise from smooth muscle

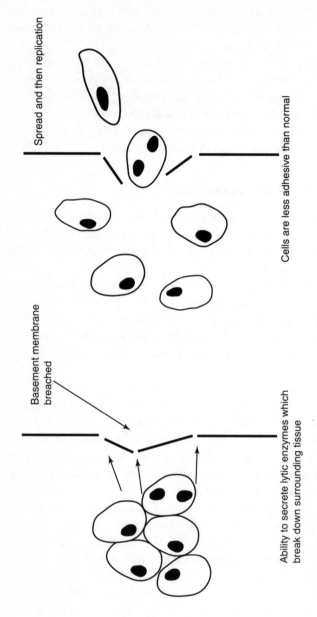

Figure 3.4 Tumour breaching basement membrane prior to infiltration.

they are called leiomyosarcomas, and if from blood vessels, haemangiosarcomas. In the benign variety, they are called, fibromas, leiomyomas, or haemangiomas respectively. A new category of tumours has been added to this list – malignant fibrous histiocytoma.

3.2 CAUSATION OF TUMOURS

Neoplasia is probably a non-specific response to a wide variety of causative agents. In this respect, it resembles chronic inflammation which is caused by infective agents, physical trauma, chemicals, and radiation. Whereas, we can identify most naturally occurring agents which cause chronic inflammation, the aetiology of cancer is obscure – to overcome this gap in our knowledge it is said that most of the tumours in man are of "spontaneous" origin. This statement really means that we are unable to identify the aetiology of most tumours seen in man or animals. There are exceptions: ionising radiation and some chemicals and viruses are carcinogenic. The former affects both man and animals but viruses mainly affect rodents, particularly mice. There is increasing evidence that they may be important in inducing cancer in larger animals and in man.

Chronic inflammation is also known to lead to the production of tumours, for example, tumours develop round the edges of varicose ulcers, in the lesions of *Lupus vulgaris* and Marjolin's ulcer. In animals, particularly in laboratory animals, a reactive response in any tissue may lead to cancer production if maintained for a long time.

3.2.1 Mechanism of tumour production

The commonly accepted view at the moment is that neoplasia arises as a result of mutagenic change brought about by chemicals, radiation, viruses, or by some "spontaneous" error of reproduction during cell division. It is probable that each agent induces more than one type of mutagenic change. Most of these are probably of no consequence, others may lead to the eventual demise of their clones, a very few may confer on the cell the property of unrestrained proliferation. This view is widely held but lacks direct experimental verification.

3.2.2 Tissue growth and cancer

Tissue growth occurs predominantly during foetal development and to compensate for tissue lost by accident or disease in extra-uterine life. Tissue growth also occurs in hormonally sensitive tissue when exposed to the appropriate hormones.

Clinical observations in man have shown that hormones, such as oestrogen, testosterone or prolactin induces hyperplasia and hypertrophy in the target organ. Two of these organs are a common site for tumour development, suggesting some causal connection. A similar situation occurs in rodents, administration of steroid hormones will produce hyperplasia in mammary tissue and if treatment is continued for a long enough period cancer will be produced. Similarly other studies revealed that the pituitary and thyroid also respond by hyperplasia in the first instance and by tumour development if treatment is prolonged.

In these experimental investigations all the compounds that induced cancer were either non-genotoxic or had hormonal activity and therefore did not cause any genetic damage. Despite this, these compounds were able to produce cancer.

Chapter 4

Immunology – an introduction

Our immune system protects us against a variety of infectious micro-organisms, such as bacteria, viruses and fungi that are found in the environment. Intact skin forms an effective barrier against invasion. However, despite our vigilance, other types of proteins and microbes can gain access through damage and penetrate mucous membranes of the lungs, nasopharynx, gastrointestinal and urogenital tracts. Once inside the body, the immune system is able to recognise these micro-organisms as foreign through its enormous variety of cells and molecules and thereby mount a response to eliminate or neutralise pathogens. Our immune system is therefore crucial to our survival. It is currently divided into two categories which are innate (non-specific) immunity and acquired (specific) immunity.

4.1 INNATE (NON-SPECIFIC) IMMUNITY

Every individual is born with a basic resistance to pathogenic micro-organisms. This resistance includes the skin as mentioned, as well as body temperature that inhibits growth of some micro-organisms, and an acidic pH of the stomach that kills ingested micro-organisms. In addition, a variety of soluble proteins, such as lysozyme and complement contribute to the innate immunity. Lysozyme are enzymes found in mucous secretions that cleave bacterial cell walls, and complement

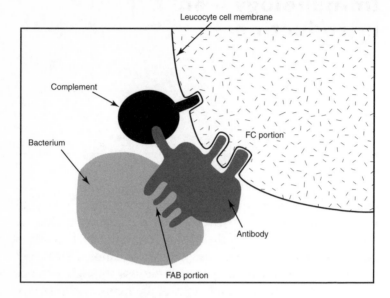

Figure 4.1 Antigen surrounded by complement and antibodies prior to lysis.

are serum proteins that bind to microbes and damage the membrane through an enzymatic cascade (Figure 4.1).

The cellular defence of the innate immune system includes cells known as phagocytes. Phagocyte literally means "to eat cells", as they are able to engulf and destroy whole pathogenic mirco-organisms. These specialised cells include blood monocytes, tissue macrophages and neutrophils. Phagocytes play a key role in eliminating micro-organisms during tissue damage where they are attracted to the site of injury by a variety of chemicals (chemotaxis). This process is part of the inflammatory response.

The innate cellular defence is non-specific as it uses recognition systems that allow cells and molecules of the immune system to bind to a variety of micro-organisms. The immune response mounted has no memory and therefore does not alter on repeated exposure.

4.2 ACQUIRED (SPECIFIC) IMMUNITY

This type of immunity is mediated when foreign molecules or micro-organisms (known as antigen) are specifically recognised by the cells of the acquired immune system (Table 4.1). These cells fall into two major groups: T-lymphocytes and B-lymphocytes. Their antigenic specificity occurs through unique antigen-binding receptors expressed on their membrane surface. These cells are produced in such a diverse number that they are capable of distinguishing different antigen by a single amino acid.

4.2.1 B-lymphocytes

The receptor on B-lymphocytes is known as membrane-bound antibody (Figure 4.2). Upon encountering antigen they rapidly divide into memory B-cells and plasma cells. Plasma cells secrete soluble antibody that bind to antigen and enhance phagocytosis. Memory B-cells have a long life-span and mount a stronger immune response on repeated exposure to the antigen.

Table 4.1 Summary of innate and acquired immunity defences

Innate immunity		Acquired immunity	
Mechanism	Response	Mechanism	Response
Skin	Non-specific	T-cells	Highly specific
Temperature	No memory	T-helper (T_H)	Possesses memory
Acidic pH of	Response	T-cytotoxic	Response improves
stomach	does not	(T_C)	on repeated
Lysozyme	alter on	B-cells	exposure
Complement	repeated	Memory B-	Diverse
Phagocytes	exposure	cells	
Inflammation		Plasma cells	

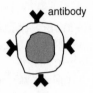

Figure 4.2 B-lymphocyte.

4.2.2   T-lymphocytes

T-lymphocytes are divided into two main subpopulations, called T-helper (T_H) cells and T-cytotoxic (T_C) cells, and are distinguished from each other by their membrane glycoproteins, CD4 and CD8 respectively (Figure 4.3). The receptor on T-lymphocytes is known as the T-cell receptor (TCR) and can only recognise antigen when they are associated with membrane proteins known as major histo-compatibility complex (MHC) molecules.

T_H cells, activated upon interacting with an antigen–MHC II molecule complex, secrete chemicals called cytokines that communicate with cells from the innate and acquired immune system to participate in the response. T_C cells are activated by an antigen–MHC I complex, resulting in destruction of antigen.

There are instances where the immune system can go wrong. Some examples are:

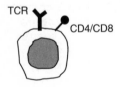

Figure 4.3 T-lymphocyte.

1   *Allergy (or hypersensitivity)*   The immune response is inappropriate or becomes exaggerated causing a heightened inflammatory response.

2   *Acquired Immunodeficiency Syndrome (AIDS)*   AIDS is acquired through the human immunodeficiency virus (HIV), where infection with the virus leave individuals susceptible to infection and certain rare forms of cancer. The virus mainly infects T_H cells as it is able to bind to the membrane glycoprotein CD_4 and infect the cell.

3   *Autoimmunity*   Although the immune system eliminates most self-reactive lymphocytes during their development, individuals still possess lymphocytes that can react to "self" cells. These lymphocytes are regulated by clonal suppression, however, the process can break down leading to autoimmunity.

The immune system is a highly organised and effective defence mechanism against invading pathogenic microorganisms. The acquired immunity and innate immunity do not operate in isolation, but complement each other to produce an overall effective and efficient immune response.

Chapter 5

Causation of disease

Disease may be classified into three major groups which are genetically determined, acquired and congenital diseases.

5.1 GENETICALLY DETERMINED

The genome is the alternative name now given to the nucleus of the mammalian cell. It is the principal repository of the genetic code and is well endowed with mechanisms for detecting any damage to it and for repairing itself if it gets damaged. The mapping out of the human genetic code will make it much easier to identify which sequences are encoded for a specific protein.

In genetically determined diseases, there is a demonstrable abnormality in the chromosomes, which is then transferred to the offspring during meiosis. Two examples illustrate:

1   Haemophilia is due to a recessive gene which when expressed leads to the impairment of blood coagulation.
2   Xeroderma pigmentosum is another example. When skin is exposed to sunlight or ultraviolet light Type B (UVB), genetic damage occurs which leads to the development of skin tumours.

5.2 ACQUIRED – INFECTIVE AGENTS

Most communicable diseases in man are caused by infective micro-organism and range from prions (a protein which behaves like a virus) to worms (an infestation – a word conventionally reserved for worms).

Viruses, bacteria and other micro-organism have the ability to invade and establish themselves in the host. Bacteria bring about their harmful effect by the production of toxin. Viruses are dependent for their harmful effects through their cytopathic potency, the type of target organ affected and the resistance of the host.

Chemicals Most chemical agents interact with animal tissues. The lesions produced may vary from those, which occur at subcellular level and therefore cannot be identified unless specialised equipment is available, (e.g. electron microscope) to those which produce overt tissue damage. Responses of this type form the subject matter of this book.

A large and important group of chemicals produce select-ive injury in a particular organ or cell type. Effects of this sort are best illustrated in the liver. This organ sits astride the portal vein and is exposed to any chemical absorbed from the intestine. It is endowed with a vast array of enzymes by means of which it carries out a vast number of complex metabolic processes. Activation of toxic or carcinogenic chemicals takes place here. A substantial proportion of these inter-mediates is excreted via the kidney, providing a reason for the proclivity of this organ to be next to the liver in its response to toxic or carcinogenic agents. Other examples of specificity are barbiturate, which in very high doses damages neurones and naphthylamine, which are specific to urothelium.

Physical agents These comprise solid objects (e.g. police-man's truncheon, knife etc.), heat, cold, electricity, ionising radiation, reduction or increase of gaseous pressure. In all instances, physical agents cause injury by the rapid transfer of energy to the target tissues.

Immunology The mammalian organisms need protection from foreign proteins. A very efficient system has been developed to counteract this danger. This system is called immunology. It is able to detect the presence of foreign proteins and to generate antibodies against them. This topic is dealt in more detail in the section on immunology.

Dietary factors Doll was one of the early workers who found evidence that lifestyle could be a cause of an increase in cancer. Others quickly followed and it gradually became clear that a high caloric diet may be the cause of an increase in cancer in various sites. There was also a higher incidence of cardiac and arteriolar disease in heavy drinkers.

Dietary deficiency, if severe, leads to malnutrition and to specific diseases e.g. Kwashiorkor. Individual components of the diet may also be a cause of disease. Thus, Fe deficiency causes anaemia, thiamine deficiency causes polyneuritis, ascorbic acid deficiency causes scurvy.

5.3 CONGENITAL DISEASE

This group of diseases develop during foetal life and may show themselves in adult life. A good example is the papilloma of the colon which starts in the gut and manifests itself in adult life. In another situation, the mother may transmit harmful agents such as Rubella virus (German measles). The disease can be fatal if infection takes place during the first three months of uterine life – causes foetal abnormalities. Likewise, a mother with HIV may transmit the virus during gestation to the offspring who may manifest the disease after birth. The mother may transmit noxious agents e.g. cigarette smoking, alcohol drinking, etc. In these examples, foetal damage occurs during gestation – but the result of this damage occurs after birth.

Chapter 6

Some recent advances in pathology

Most teachers of pathology start by defining pathology as a science of disease. Very good, but what is science. The word science is derived from the Latin word *scire* to learn, to know, and is applied to the acquisition of knowledge. This process involves a number of logical steps, which can be formulated as:

1   statement of the problem;
2   generation of a hypothesis;
3   observation and experimentation;
4   results and interpretation; and
5   conclusion.

Taken together they are called the scientific method.

This method helps us to discover facts, which are then placed in order according to certain rules, which are called laws. The laws of science are different from the laws enacted by Parliament or some other legislative body. If anyone breaks a civil law, one is liable for punishment but the law remains intact. If a law in science is broken by a new discovery then the law is invalid and a new one will take its place.

Examples of this type of science are chemistry, physics, astronomy, and thermodynamics and these are known as basic sciences. Pathology has no laws. It has recurrent phenomena, which could act as a substitute.

Pathology employs freely the scientific method but the terms employed and results obtained are unlike those obtained from the basic sciences. These are largely based on measurements whereas pathology examines the meaning of words, analyses concepts and is continually searching for principles. This distinction can be better understood if one considers that the results from basic sciences are by and large quantitative and objective whereas, the pathology results are largely descriptive and subjective. This subjective element can be disciplined over the years to conform to a general rule – acquisition of experience. In its present form is pathology able to withstand the onslaught of molecular biology? The reader is left to draw his/her own conclusions.

6.1   RECURRENT THEMES IN PATHOLOGY

Pathology has no laws in the sense of laws in the basic sciences but it has recurrent themes – here are some examples:

Theme 1   A protective mechanism may become deranged and act as a source of disease. For example if a blood vessel is cut, thrombosis develops quickly at the site of haemorrhage forming a "plug" which prevents further bleeding. If, however, thrombosis occurs in the vessels of the heart it may result in sudden death. In autoimmune disease the antibodies, which are meant to protect the organism from foreign proteins, attack the proteins of the host.

Theme 2   The mammalian organism often overreacts to potentially damaging agents (e.g. allergic reaction, leucocytosis in some disease states).

Theme 3   Under natural conditions, a duel between host and parasite is never fought to a finish – some survive and are the source of a fresh resistant generation of organisms. For example, on the introduction of a new antibiotic, a few organisms escape the lethal effects and act as a source of resistant organisms. The same may occur with chemotherapeutic agents. Survival of some humans in epidemics is another manifestation of the same phenomenon.

Theme 4 Failure of adaptation is self reinforcing – "one damn thing follows another" e.g. cirrhosis of the liver and chronic heart disease are progressive pathological conditions ending in death.

6.2 APOPTOSIS

The morphological appearance of cell necrosis caused by toxins has been established for several decades and is well known to pathologists and cytologists. They have also recognised a type of necrosis, which is distinct from the one caused by toxins, and called it shrinking necrosis, necrobiosis, or single cell necrosis. Kerr *et al.* (*Brit. J. Cancer* 1972) embarked on a different tack. They thought that in this lesion the loss of cells was a gentle process like the falling of leaves from deciduous trees in the autumn. They borrowed a term from the Greek language – apoptosis – to describe this phenomenon.

Robert Horvitz (*The Cell* 1986) later showed that specific genes expressed in nematodes *C. elegans*, caused targeted cells to die in a regular process – programmed cell death (PCD). In fact, PCD showed many features of apoptosis identified by Kerr *et al.* in several tissues so that apoptosis was established as a synonym for PCD.

This discovery was followed by a complete turn around in the way biological research workers look at apoptosis and resulted in a massive increase in research on PCD, and there are little signs of its abating.

Since the late 1980s, the term apoptosis has been accepted in pathology to mean PCD. It differs from necrosis produced by external agents. Apoptosis is regarded as physiological – the cell dies "on cue" according to a programme in the modelling of tissues particularly during organogenesis.

At EM level, the first change is a condensation of chromatin into dense lumps at the periphery of the nucleus. Cell surface features, such as cell/cell junctions for example, gradually disappear so that the plasma membrane becomes very smooth. The cell begins to shrink due to loss of water and the organelles (mitochondria, lysosomes) become crowded. Subsequently the neighbouring cells remove the apoptotic fragments by ingesting them and break them up in their lysosomal system.

6.3 ADAPTATION

In the Introduction, disease was defined as loss of adaptation – changes with which the cell cannot cope. Clinical and veterinary practices provide some examples. Athletes undergoing intensive exercise place a considerable load on the heart above the normal levels. The heart responds by first enlarging and then by increasing the thickness of the myocardium. These changes are the new load, which the heart has to bear.

Other examples can be cited from toxicology. Thus feeding rats and mice a relatively low dose of phenobarbitone results in hepatic increase in the activity of enzyme involved in its metabolism. If the doses are gradually increased the liver enlarges in a dose – related manner and then enlargement of centrilobular cells occurs. Upto this moment, the hepatocytes have coped with the increases – further dosing results in cloudy swelling or vacuolar dilatation and eventually nodular hyperplasia. Other examples can be cited from several groups of compounds e.g. peroxisome proliferators, organochlorines and butylated hydroxytoluene (BHT), a widely used antioxidant, behave in the same way as the group of chemicals cited. It would appear that adaptation lies in the borderland between the normal cell and the affected cell.

Toxicity – Damage to the cell – may range from a mild damage to lethal.

6.4   TARGET ORGAN TOXICITY

Observation of the site of injury over many years established that the damage produced by chemicals is not a random event. Repeated administration of the same chemical by the same route, and delivered at the same site, for the same species, produce the same type of injury at the same delivery site (target). It must be pointed out that the same compound may have three or more target organs but this is a rarity.

A good example of this property of toxins is that of dimethyl nitrosamine (DMN). Nasal and hepatic damage occurs in rats when this compound is given orally. Long term administration results in the development of malignant tumours at those sites. Thus DMN has two target sites. A large number of chemicals from different chemical classes behave in much the same way as DMN.

Advances in biochemistry and molecular biology have made it possible to provide some explanation for these modes of action. Biochemical investigations have shown that DMN is metabolised by the cytochrome family of enzymes to damage DNA. The same set of enzymes are found in the nasal mucosa thus providing a plausible explanation for the close similarity of the tissue response.

6.5   ONCOGENES

Oncogenes are involved in the synthesis of proteins which involved in normal growth regulation and are bound to membranes either in the nucleus or in the cytoplasm.

There are three classes of normal regulatory genes:

1　growth promoting protooncogene;
2　growth inhibiting cancer suppressor gene; and
3　gene regulating programmed cell death (apoptosis).

6.5.1　Other genetic activity

DNA repair gene – affects carcinogenesis indirectly by influencing the ability of the organism to repair non-lethal cell damage.

Carcinogenesis is a multistep process at the molecular level progression results from the accumulation of genetic lesions tolerated by defects in DNA repair. This activity is normally under control but it can be permanently "switched on" by point mutations, gene amplification, chromosomal translocation and chromosomal rearrangement.

Chapter 7

Clinical chemistry

To gain a fuller appreciation of the toxicological significance of chemically induced histopathological changes in an organ, it is helpful to have an understanding of changes in the biochemistry and physiological function at the target site following chemical exposure. These biochemical changes are often reflected in deviation from normal levels of constituents derived from the target organ present either in the circulating blood or excreted in the urine. The measurement of these biochemical constituents gives useful evidential clues of the onset, progress and repair of chemical injury in the intact animal. This information is of value in the design of toxicological studies for the risk assessment of a chemical in experimental animals and in the extrapolation of animal data to man. Furthermore, the experimental design requires a fuller understanding of the route of exposure, the absorption, distribution, metabolism and excretion of the test compound and the cascade of biochemical changes set in train in the target organ following chemical insult.

The aim of this chapter is specifically to complement the histopathological changes as described in Chapter 1 *et seq*. The text is therefore directed to identifying some of the important biochemical constituents in the circulating blood and in the urine that are of diagnostic value in indicating which target organ is likely to be adversely affected following chemical exposure. The text has been deliberately pitched at a level considered to be appropriate for readers with a superficial knowledge of mammalian biochemistry by limiting the use of technical terms to an irreducible minimum. A list of books for further reading is given at the end of the book. This chapter is divided into the following sections:

1   Enzymes: Classes of enzymes in mammalian cells and their intracellular locations; the mixed function oxidase (MFO); enzyme system mediating the bioactivation and detoxification of foreign compounds; factors influencing the induction and inhibition of MFO enzymes; soluble enzymes in body fluids of diagnostic value.

2   Proteins: Examples of proteins and polypeptides in plasma, their origin and diagnostic value in indicating tissue injury.

3   Hormones and Steroids: Examples and their location.

4   Clinical chemistry: Examples of biochemical changes in body fluid indicative of target organ toxicity. Examples of chemicals known to produce toxic effects at target sites.

5   Methodologies: Estimation of biochemical constituents in biological fluids. Assessment of human chemical exposure.

7.1   ENZYMES

7.1.1   Nature and function

Enzymes are complex high molecular weight specialised proteins of tertiary structure which are produced and occur in mammalian cells or are secreted by cells. They function as biological catalysts capable of effecting well characterised biochemical metabolic transformation reactions on ingested nutrients and other endogenously formed intermediate compounds to enable the various organs and tissues in the body to perform their specialised functions and thereby, to ensure the viability and well being of the mammalian host.

Additionally, mammalian enzyme systems have the ability of mediating the biotransformation of many exogenous substances that man is deliberately or inadvertently exposed to, such as drugs, additives and contaminants in the human diet, industrial chemicals and environmental pollutants.

These complex protein entities, either present bound to cellular membranes (desmoenzymes) or as free soluble enzymes (lysoenzymes), catalyzing a wide and diverse range of biochemical reactions are characterised by having specific areas of active sites on the enzyme to which substrates bind. The enzyme–substrate complexes become activated and the reaction products are formed on the surface of the enzyme. The products are then released from the enzyme allowing the active sites to bind more substrate molecules for processing. Thus, enzyme activity is characterised by the binding affinity of substrate molecules to the active sites on the surface of an enzyme and the rate at which the enzyme catalyses the reaction (the turnover number i.e. the number of molecules of substrate transformed per minute). By common agreement, enzymes are now generally named by adding the suffix -ase either to the substrate (e.g. glucosidase) or to a phrase describing the catalytic reaction mediated by the enzyme (e.g. glucose oxidase). The few exceptions to this general rule are proteins such as trypsin, renin, pepsin and cathepsin, which for historical reasons have remained unchanged.

7.1.2 Enzyme classification

Mammalian enzymes have been grouped into six main classes by the International Union of Biochemistry and Molecular Biology (IUBMB). The six main classes based on the general types of enzymic reactions catalysed are: (1) oxido-reductases; (2) transferases; (3) hydrolases; (4) isomerases; (5) lyases; and (6) ligases. The main classes of enzyme activities are further divided into sub-classes and these are summarised in Table 7.1.

Table 7.1 International classification of enzymes and major sub-classes

Major class	Sub-classes
Oxido-reductases	Dehydrogenases Oxidases Reductases Peroxidases Catalase Oxygenases Hydroxylases
Hydrolases	Esterases Glycosidases Peptidases Thiolases Phophatases Phospholipases Amidases Deaminases Ribonucleases
Isomerases	Racemases Epimerases Isomerases Mutases (not all)
Transferases	Transaldolases Transketolases Aceyl-, Methyl-, Glucosyl-, sulpho- and Phosphoryl-transferases
Lyases	Decarboxylases Aldolases Hydratases Dehydratases Synthases Lyases
Ligases	Synthetases Carboxylases

Source: IUBMB.

7.1.3 Intracellular location

Enzymes are located at various sites within a mammalian cell, ranging from the outer plasma membrane to the nucleus. Their primary function at a particular site or organelle is to carry out the biochemical transformation reaction for which they are uniquely designed, and participate in the process of metabolic degradation or the synthesis of endogenous substances, intended either for use by the cell or for export. Thus, the main enzymes in the plasma membrane participate in the internalisation of nutrients and elements required for maintaining the viability of the cell, such as amino acids, glucose, fatty acids and essential inorganic elements, and in the export of intracellularly produced substances, like albumin, globulins and lipids, into the circulating blood. The nucleus, the main repository of the genetic character of the cell contains enzyme systems involved in the biosynthesis of DNA and RNA. Table 7.2 summarises the intracellular location of various enzymes.

Many of the enzymic reactions are energy dependent processes requiring the expenditure of energy to drive the reaction forward. The common fuel used in these processes is adenosine triphosphate (ATP) produced by the controlled combustion of glucose in the mitochondria. Thus, the mitochondria are replete with enzymes involved in the metabolic degradation of glucose. The first process involves the anaerobic glycolysis of the 6-carbon containing sugar to 3-carbon intermediates followed by the enzymic degradation of these intermediates to carbon dioxide by the action of enzymes of the tricarboxylic acid cycle pathway. This catabolic process leads to the synthesis of ATP, the common currency in the body enabling biological reactions requiring the expenditure of energy to function. Other biochemical reactions carried out in the mitochondria include the β-oxidation of fatty acid, amino acid oxidation, fatty acid elongation, and urea synthesis.

Other organelles containing enzymes with special functional roles are the lysosomes and peroxisomes. Lysosomes contain a variety of hydrolytic enzymes whose specific function

Table 7.2 Intracellular location of some major enzyme systems in mammalian metabolism pathways (also included are some enzymes in the G.I. Microflora)

Plasma membrane	Cholinesterases, Catalase, Triosephosphate dehydrogenase, Adenosine triphosphatases (ATPases), NADase
Cytoplasm	Glycolysis: hexose monophosphate pathway, Glycogenesis and glycogenolysis, Fatty acid synthesis, Purine and pyrimidine catabolism, Peptidases, Aminotransferases, Amino acyl synthetases
Mitochondria	Tricarboxylic acid cycle, Fatty acid oxidation, Amino acid oxidation, Fatty acid elongation, Urea synthesis, Electron transport and coupled phosphorylation
Lysosomes	Lysozyme, Acid phosphatase, Hydrolases – including proteases, lipase, nucleases, glycosidases, aryl sulphatases, phospholipases and phophatases
Peroxisomes	Urate oxidase, D-amino acid oxidase, α-hydroxy acid oxidase, long-chain fatty acid oxidase
Endoplasmic reticulum	NADH- and NADPH-cytochrome c reductase, Cytochrome b_5 and cytochrome P-450 Mixed Function Oxidases (MFO) enzyme system, glucose-6-phosphatase, nucleoside diphosphatase, esterases, glucuronidases, glucuronyltransferases, protein synthetic pathways, steroid synthesis and reduction, phosphoglyceride and triacyl glycerol synthesis
Golgi apparatus	Galactosyl- and glucosyltransferase, chondroitin sulfotransferase, 5'-nucleotidase, NADH-cytochrome c reductase, glucose-6-phosphatase
Nucleus	DNA and RNA biosynthetic pathways
Gastro-intestinal microflora	Ester and Amide Hydrolases, N- and O-Dealkylases, Reductases, Aromatases

is to engulf, scavenge and clear by hydrolytic action the debris resulting from injury to organelles, that is, to act as a "suicide" squad. Peroxisomes, generally sparsely present in the liver and other organs, contain enzymes mediating among other reactions, the oxidation of uric acid and the omega-oxidation of long-chain fatty acids. This organelle has attracted considerable attention in recent years as a variety of compounds including a number of hypolipidaemic drugs and esters of ortho-phthalic acid used as plasticisers and solvents, have been found to induce peroxisome proliferation in rodent livers. The proliferation of this organelle in the rodent liver has been associated with the development of liver tumours.

The ER, consisting of rough ER and smooth ER, constitute an important organelle in the synthesis of endogenous proteins and in the metabolic biotransformation of foreign compounds. The biochemical fraction obtained by the differential centrifugation of tissue homogenates, known as the microsomal fraction, contains both rough and smooth ER. Ribosomes in the rough ER are the site for protein synthesis. They contain two subunits that combine with mRNA and various enzymes to form the "factory" for the production of proteins. The rough ER contains a high concentration of electron transport proteins, glucose-6-phosphatase and ATPase activity.

Smooth ER occurs in the cell in intimate contact with mitochondria and contains high levels of the haemoproteins cytochrome b_5 and cytochrome P-450. Enzymes associated with cytochrome P-450, collectively referred to as the mixed function oxidase (MFO) enzyme system play an important role in the metabolic transformation of foreign compounds. The range and types of biotransformation reactions mediated by the MFO enzymes and other mammalian enzyme system will be described in next section. Other enzyme activities present in the smooth ER include monoamine oxidase, NAD(P)H-cytochrome c reductase, nucleotide diphosphatase, esterase, aldolase, and glutamine synthetase.

The cytoplasm contains a wide range of soluble enzymes involved in metabolic processes of importance in the catabolism of glycogen, sugars, protein, purine and pyrimidine, and also in the synthesis of glycogen and fatty acids (see Table 7.2). Many of these cytosolic enzymes leak across the plasma membrane in small quantities into the circulation blood and other body fluids in normal conditions. However, in the event of tissue damage involving the disruption of plasma membrane integrity, these enzymes leak in substantial amounts into the circulation and their measurement provides valuable clues as to the site of internal injury. The enzymes present in the serum found to be of particular diagnostic value in indicating the site of tissue damage are shown in Table 7.3.

The activity of an enzyme, as a measure of its level, in the circulation under normal conditions depends on a balance between the rates of synthesis of the enzyme in the tissue and of its release into blood on the one hand, and on the other, on the clearance rate of the enzyme from circulation. Following tissue damage resulting either from a pathological

Table 7.3 Serum enzymes of diagnostic value indicative of tissue injury

Enzyme	Origin
Acid phosphatase	Prostate, Erythrocytes
Alanine aminotransferase (ALT)	Liver
Alkaline phosphatase (ALP)	Hepatobiliary tree, Bone, GI tract, Kidney
Amylase	Pancreas, Salivary glands
Aspartate aminotransferase (AST)	Liver, Heart muscle, Skeletal muscle
Cholinesterase	Liver
Creatine kinase (CK)	Skeletal muscle, Heart muscle, Brain
Gamma-Glutamyl Transferase (GGT)	Liver, Pancreas
Lactate dehydrogenase (LDH)	Liver, Cardiac muscle, Skeletal muscle

process or from chemical injury, the rate of entry of the marker enzyme into the circulation is greatly increased and its measurement provides useful supportive evidence to the clinical picture in identifying the site of damage.

7.1.4 Enzymes involved in xenobiotic metabolism

Foreign chemicals entering the body following exposure by inhalation, skin absorption, ingestion or by the parenteral routes are metabolised by a wide variety of enzyme systems. Table 7.4 shows examples of a number of enzymic processes mediating biotransformation reactions on foreign chemicals in mammalian systems. The endoplasmic reticulum where the MFO enzymes, centred on the haemoprotein cytochrome P-450 are located, constitute an important group of enzymes mediating both bioactivation and detoxification reactions on foreign chemicals. These reactions are collectively classed as Phase 1 reactions. Additionally, the ER contains enzymes capable of further metabolising the Phase 1 reaction metabolites to more water-soluble glucuronide and sulphate conjugated products (Phase 2 reactions). Enzymes of the MFO system are found in most organs but the major site is the liver. Other organs containing toxicologically significant amounts of the MFO system, albeit to a smaller extent than in the liver, are the cortex in kidneys, in the epidermal layer of skin, in type 11 pneumocytes and Clara cells in the lung and in the adrenal cortex, much smaller amounts have been found in the small intestine, in the testes and ovaries, and in the placenta.

The metabolic biotransformation fate of a compound leading either to the lethal synthesis of a toxic metabolite or to the formation of a non-toxic product may be summarised as follows:

In the scheme depicted in Figure 7.1 if Compound X is toxic *per se*, Pathway A may operate to detoxify it. If Compound X is non-toxic, metabolism may proceed either by Pathway A or

Table 7.4 Enzymic processes mediating the metabolic bioactivation and detoxification of foreign compounds

Enzymic reaction	Chemical class	Examples
Hydrolysis	carboxylic acid esters	Acetyl salicylic acid, Pethidine, Pyrethroids, Carbamates, Dialkyl phthalates and Adipates
	carboxyl acid amides	Phenacetin, Penicillin, Carbanilates
	Glucuronides	Phenolphthalein glucuronide
	Glycosides	Cycasin, Amygdalin, Thioglyosides
	Aryl sulphates	Steroid sulphates
Oxidation (MFO system)	Aromatic hydroxylation	Benzene, Aromatic hydrocarbons
	Aromatic epoxidation	Acetanilide
	Aliphatic hydroxylation	Alkanes, Fatty acids
	O-dealkylation	Codeine, Phenacetin
	S-dealkylation	Methyl mercaptan, Methylisothiourea
	S-oxidation	Carbon disulphide, Parathion
	N-oxidation	Hydroxylamine, 2-acetylamino fluorene
	N-hydroxylation	Dimethylaniline, Morphine
	De-sulphuration	Parathion
	De-halogenation	Halothane, DDT
	N-dealkylation	t-amines, Amphetamine
Oxidation (mediated by dehydrogenases and oxidases)	Alcohol → Aldehyde	Ethanol, allyl alcohol
	Aldehyde → Acid	Formaldehyde,
	Amines → Aldehyde	Tolualdehyde Tryptamine, Tyramine
Reductions (MFO system)	Polycyclic arene oxide reduction	Benzo(a)pyrene-4, 5-oxide

	Azo compounds → amines	Prontosil, Butter yellow
	Nitro compounds → amines	Nitrobenzene, Chloramphenicol
	N-oxide → tertiary amine	Nicotine-N-oxide, Indacine-N-oxide
	Aryl and alkylhalide dehalogenation	DDT, Trichloro-fluoromethane
Reduction (mediated by dehydrogenases and reductases)	Carbonyl reduction	Cyclohexanone, Benzaldehyde, p-Nitroacetophenone, Chloral hydrate

Conjugations (mediated by UDP-glucuronyl transferases)

Glucuronic acid conjugation with:	Aryl and alkyl alcohols	Phenol, Propane-1,2-diol, Sterols
	Primary/Secondary amines	Aniline, Sulphonamides, N-hydroxyarylamines
	Sulphydric compounds	Thiophenols
	Carboxylic acids	Phenylacetic acid, other arylacetic acids, Carbamic acids

Conjugations (mediated by Sulphotransferases, Amino acid N-acyl transferases, Methyl transferases, Glutathione-S-transferases, Acyl-CoA: aminotransferase)

Sulphate conjugation with:	Phenols	Phenol
	Aromatic amines	2-Acetylaminofluorene
	Alkanols	Oestradiol and other sterols
Glutathione conjugation with:	Arene and alkene oxides	Styrene-7,8-oxide, Benzo(a)pyrene-4, 5-oxide
Amino acid (e.g. Glycine) conjugation with:	Carboxylic acids	Benzoic acid, Salicylic acid, Cinnamic acid

Table 7.4 (Continued)

Enzymic reaction	Chemical class	Examples
O- and N-Methylation reactions with:		Phenols, Catechol, Imidazole, Histamine
Phosphotransferases Phosphate conjugation with:		Phenol

Pathway B or by an interplay of the two pathways, the latter pathway leading to the formation of toxic reactive intermediates. The interactive balance of enzymic reactions of these two pathways on Compound X eventually determines the metabolic fate of Compound X in the body and whether or not a toxic effect would result at a target site.

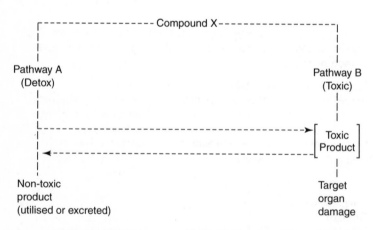

Figure 7.1 Bioactivation and detoxification scheme for foreign chemicals.

It must be emphasised that the above biotransformation reactions scheme is an oversimplified version of the much more complex sequence of metabolic events encountered by a foreign chemical in the living mammalian system. A detailed understanding of the ultimate metabolic and toxicological fate of a foreign compound in the body requires physiologically-based pharmacokinetic (PBPK) studies to be carried on a test compound generating data on the absorption, metabolism, disposition, retention and excretion of the compound in the body and information on the dosimetry of the compound (that is, the effective dose of the compound or its reactive metabolites at the target site).

7.1.5 Structural variants of enzymes and cytochrome P-450 haemoprotein polymorphisms

Multiple forms of an enzyme with similar catalytic action but with different physico-chemical characteristics, known as isoenzymes, have been found to be of particular value is distinguishing the tissue source of enzymes in the circulation. Isoenzyme variants have been characterised by differences in electrophoretic mobilities, immunochemical properties and differential enzyme–substrate affinity and catalytic activity. Examples of isoenzymes of diagnostic value in Clinical Chemistry are lactate dehydrogenase (LDH) and creatine kinase (CK). Five isoenzymes of LDH have been identified in serum and of these LDH (H_4) originates from the heart and LDH (M_4) from the liver. In the case of CK which consists of three isoenzymes (1) originating from the heart; (2) skeletal muscle; or (3) the brain, CK(MB) originates from heart muscle, CK(MM) from skeletal muscle and CK(BB) from the brain. The measurement of these CK isoenzymes in serum indicates its tissue source.

It has become increasingly clear that the susceptibility of individuals to adverse health effects following exposure to a chemical is influenced by the balance between bioactivating and detoxifying enzymic processes and the complement of enzymes mediating these two processes are under genetic control. Thus, toxicity is to a significant extent influenced by the genetic makeup of an individual. The MFO system intensively studied in this context has revealed that "Cytochrome P-450" is not a single haemoprotein but comprises a superfamily of haemoproteins each with an identical prosthetic group, but different apoprotein structures, which are responsible for different substrate specificities. Currently, at least 27 families with up to eight subfamilies and up to 23 individual forms have been identified. Many of these families are present in all mammals including man. Examples of some of the main isoforms of the haemoprotein and the substrates metabolised are shown in Table 7.5. The table also shows some of the chemicals known to induce or inhibit enzyme reaction mediated by the isoforms of cytochrome P-450. Many independent studies have now confirmed the importance of phenotypic polymorphisms in foreign chemical metabolism as risk factors in the development of cancers and other toxic effects in experimental animals and in man following chemical exposure. Early evidence for polymorphism came from metabolic studies on phenacetin, mediated by the enzymic activity of the isoform CYP1A1, which showed a 58-fold variation in the O-dealkylation of the compound in different human subjects. A similar range of variation in CYP1A1 activity in humans, as measured by caffeine 3-demethylation, has been demonstrated. Considerable interindividual variability has also been found with respect to human liver N-oxidation of 2-naphthylamine and 2-acetylaminofluorene.

7.2   PROTEINS IN PLASMA

In addition to enzymes derived from various organs and tissues, a wide variety of proteins are found in the plasma fraction of blood. Table 7.6 shows some of the important

Table 7.5 Isoforms of the Cytochrome P-450 superfamily mediating mixed function oxidase reactions

Subfamily/ Protein	Inducers	Inhibitors	Substrates
1A			
1A1	3-MC, TCDD, ARO	9-HE, α-NF	7-Ethoxyresorufin
1A2	3-MC, ISO, TCDD	9-HE, α-NF	Caffeine, Acetanilide
2A			
2A1	PB, 3-MC, PCN	–	Coumarin, Testosterone
2A2	Non-inducible	–	–
2B			
2B1	PB, Ethanol, DEX	SB, SKF-525A	Pentoxyresorufin
2B2	PB, ARO, PCN, DEX	–	Benzphetamine
2B4	PB	–	–
2D			
2D1	Non-inducible	Ajamalicine, Quinidine	Debrisoquine
2E			
2E1	Ethanol, DMSO, Isoniazid	Diallyl sulphide	4-Nitrophenol, Nitrosodimethylamine
3A			
3A1	PCN, PB, DEX	Erythromycin	Testosterone
3A2	PB	–	Testosterone
3A4	PB, DEX	17-Ethynyl-oestradiol	Nifedipine
3A6	RIF	–	–
4A			
4A1	CLOF	Terminal acetylinic fatty acids	Lauric acid

3-MC = 3-methylcholanthrene; 9-HE = 9-hydroxyellipticine; α-NF = α-naphthoflavone; ARO = Arochlor 1254; CLOF = clofibrate; DEX = dexamethasone; DMSO = dimethyl-sulphoxide; ISO = isosafrole; PB = phenobarbitone; PCN = pregenolone-16-α-carbonitrile; RIF = rifampicin; TCDD = 2,3,7,8-tetrachlorodibenzodioxin.

Table 7.6 Examples of proteins in plasma of potential diagnostic value for monitoring disease

Protein	Principal function	Used for diagnosing
Pre-albumin	Transport function (?)	Liver disease, malnutrition
Albumin	Colloid oncotic pressure, Transport function	Liver, kidney and GI disease
α_1-Globulins		
Fetoprotein	Unknown	Neural tube defects, Marker for tumours
Protease inhibitor (API)	Antiprotease	Lung and liver disease (API deficiency due to genetic polymorphism)
Prothrombin	Blood clotting	Coagulation screen, Liver function test
α_2-Globulins		
Ceruloplasmin	Copper transport	Wilson's disease, malnutrition
Haptoglobin	Haemoglobin	Haemolytic disorders
Macroglobulin	Antiprotease, transport functions	Proteinuria
Thyroxine-binding globulin	T_4 and T_3 transport	Thyroid disease
β-Globulins		
C-Reactive protein	Body's defence mechanisms	Considered to be involved in response to foreign materials
β_2-Microglobulin	Body's defence mechanisms	Renal failure, monitoring myeloma
Transferrin	Iron transport	Iron deficiency
γ-Globulins (IgG, IgA, Igm etc.)	Body's defence mechanisms	Liver disease, Auto-immune disease
Troponins- (T, C, I)	Regulatory complex in tropomyosin strands in muscle	Troponins T and I – markers of myocardial infarction

proteins present, their principal functions and their use in the diagnosis of various disease conditions in humans.

Most plasma proteins are synthesised in the liver, with the exception of immunoglobulins by lymphocytes, apolipoproteins by enterocytes, β_2-microglobulin which is a cell surface protein and the troponins present in muscles. It is estimated that in humans about 25 g of plasma proteins are synthesised daily and secreted into the circulation there being no mechanism for intracellular storage.

The main functions of plasma proteins include the transport in the blood of various vitamins (Vitamin A), essential elements (calcium, iron and copper), cholesterol, triglycerides and hormones (thyroxine and tri-iodothyronine; T_4 and T_3 respectively), the maintenance of plasma oncotic pressure, buffering pH changes, conferring humoral immunity, facilitate clotting and respond to acute inflammatory reactions.

Thus for example, following trauma, infections, inflammation, etc. the body responds by initiating a series of mechanisms leading to increased plasma levels of C-reactive protein, anti-protease inhibitors, ceruloplasmin, the haptoglobins and α_1-acid glycoprotein. The cytokines and a host of vasoactive substances, such as prostaglandins and histamine, are important mediators of the acute-phase response.

A number of proteins in plasma have been found to be useful markers for the diagnosis of tumours and for monitoring the effects of treatment and prognosis. These are shown in Table 7.7.

Other markers found to be of value are catecholamines and their metabolites in phaeochromocytoma and serotonin (5-hydroxytrytamine) derived from tryptophan, and its metabolite 5-hydroxyindole acetic acid (5-HIAA) in carcinoid tumours. However, it must be stated that, in general, tumour markers are not specific enough and of limited value in screening for asymptomatic disease. In certain specific instances tumour markers may be used to screen for high-risk groups. Examples include measuring calcitonin after pentagastrin

Table 7.7 Examples of plasma proteins as markers of tumours

Plasma protein marker	Malignancy
Human chorionic gonadotropin (hCG)	Choriocarcinoma, Germ Cell
Carcinoembryonic antigen (CEA)	Colorectal
Prostate specific antigen (PSA)	Prostate
Calcitonin	Thyroid (medullary)
Thyroglobulin	Thyroid (follicular)
Paraprotein (monoclonal immunoglobulins)	Multiple myeloma
Bence-Jones Proteins in urine	Multiple myeloma

stimulation to screen close relatives of patients with medullary carcinoma of the thyroid and the measurement of human chorionic gonadotropin (hCG) to screen for choriocarcinoma in women who have had a hydatidiform mole. Tumour markers can only be used for prognosis on the few occasions when the plasma concentration of the marker correlates with the tumour mass. Thus, for example hCG is used in choriocarcinoma, immunoglobin G (IgG) in paraproteinaemia, and alpha-fetoprotein (AFP) and hCG in testicular tumours.

7.3   HORMONES AND STEROIDS IN PLASMA

The cascade of activity of the hypothalamic-pituitary-adrenal axis provides the pivotal stimuli for the production and control of hormones by the various organs of the endocrine system in the body. The hypothalamus on being stimulated by neurotransmitters controlled by the central nervous system (CNS), releases several regulatory factors into the blood supplying the anterior pituitary where they control and regulate the synthesis and secretion of hormones into the circulation. Generally, there are two feedback loops controlling the synthesis of hormones. In the long feedback loop, the final hormone binds receptors on the cells of the anterior pituitary gland, the hypothalamus and the CNS to prevent further elaboration of hormones from those cells that are involved in the cascade. The short feedback loop is accounted for by the pituitary hormone that feeds back negatively on the hypothalamus operating through a cognate receptor. These mechanisms provide tight controls on the operation of the cascade responding to stimulating signals and also to inhibitory feedback systems. Table 7.8 lists some of the hypothalamus releasing hormones and their stimulatory or inhibitory effects on anterior pituitary hormone production.

The polypeptide hormones secreted by the anterior pituitary gland include growth hormone (GH) responsible for regulat-

Table 7.8 Examples of some hypothalamic releasing hormones and their effects on anterior pituitary hormone production

Hypothalamus releasing hormone	Anterior pituitary hormone released or inhibited
Thyrotropin releasing hormone (TRH)	Thyrotropin (TSH) released; Can also release Prolactin experimentally
Gonadotropin releasing hormone (GnRH)	Lactogenic hormone (LH) and Follicle-stimulating hormone (FSH) released
Gonadotropin release inhibiting factor (GnRIF)	LH and FSH release inhibited
Corticotropin releasing hormone (CRH)	ACTH and some β-endorphin released
Arginine vasopressin (AVP)	Stimulates CRH action in ACTH released Releases ACTH with 5-HT
Angiotensin II (AII)	Stimulates CRH action in ACTH release
Somatocrinin (GRH)	Growth hormone (GH) release
Somatostatin (GIH)	GH release inhibited
Prolactin releasing factor (PRF)	Releases prolactin (PRL)
Prolactin release inhibiting factor (PIF)	Inhibits PRL release

ing bone and body tissue growth and carbohydrate and protein metabolism, thyrotropin or thyroid stimulating hormone (TSH) acting on the thyroid controls the production of triiodothyronine (T_3) and thyroxine (T_4), adrenocorticotropic hormone (ACTH) responsible for steroid hormones production by the adrenal cortex and catecholamines by the inner medulla, β-lipotropin (β-LTH) mediating β-endorphin synthesis, corticotropin-like intermediary peptide (CLIP) stimulating insulin release from β-cells of the pancreas in the presence of glucose, prolactin (PRL) acting on the mammary glands to stimulate milk synthesis, and follicle-stimulating hormone (FSH) and luteinizing hormone (LH) responsible for the synthesis of male and female sex hormones and for regulating gonadal function. Table 7.9 presents a list of endocrine derived substances in the blood which have been shown to be of diagnostic value for revealing endocrinal dysfunction and for identifying the target organ affected.

7.4 BIOCHEMICAL CHANGES RELATED TO CHEMICAL TOXICITY

Sections 7.1–7.3 had provided a brief overview of the various proteins, enzymes and hormones synthesised by a number of important organ systems in the body and measurable in the circulation. The concentration at which each of these endogenous substances is present in body fluid in an healthy individual is regulated and influenced by their rate of synthesis, rate of entry and removal from the circulation and fluid volume. Under normal physiological conditions their levels in body fluids of experimental animals and in humans range over narrow limits.

In circumstances where this homeostatic regulatory mechanism is compromised, either by nutritional inadequacy or the imbalance in the availability of essential nutrients, by disease states or resulting from chemically mediated toxicity to an organ system, the biosyntheses of these endogenous

Table 7.9 Examples of some endocrine derived substances of diagnostic value

Endocrine organ	Hormones and other substances
Thyroid	Thyroxine (T$_4$), Tri-iodothyronine (T$_3$), Thyrotropine (TSH)
Hypothalamo-pituitary-adrenal axis	
Hypothalamic releasing hormones	Thyrotropin releasing hormone Gonadotropin releasing hormone Corticotropin releasing hormone Prolactin releasing factor (PRF) Arginine vasopressin (AVP) Angiotensin II (AII) Somatocrinin (GRH) Somatostatin (GIH) Gastrin releasing peptide
Pituitary hormones	Growth hormone (GH) Thyrotropin (TSH) Adrenocorticotrophic hormone (ACTH) Prolactin (PRL) Follicle-stimulating hormone (FSH) Luteinizing hormone (LH)
Adrenals	Cortisol, corticosterone, Aldosterone, Androstenedione Dehydroepiandrosterone (DHEA)
Reproductive system	
Male	Androgen Binding Protein Testosterone
Female	Oestradiol, Progesterone
Pancreas	Insulin, Amylase, Lipase

substances are altered with consequent changes in their levels in the circulation. The monitoring of these changes in the intact animal provides a useful insight on the pathogenesis in an affected organ and also information on the progression or repair of tissue injury.

Some of the important mammalian organ systems liable to be damaged either by the deliberate or inadvertent exposure of the host to chemicals are the liver, the renal system, the cardio-vascular system, organs of the endocrine system, for example, the thyroid, the pancreas and the hypothalamus-pituitary-adrenal axis controlling the synthesis and release of various polypeptides regulating diverse endocrine functions. A brief description of major changes in the body fluid levels of a number of biochemical constituents reflecting adverse toxic reactions in these organs are as follows:

Liver The liver plays a vital role in the metabolism of ingested carbohydrates, proteins and amino acids, and lipids. Additionally, the liver is the important site for the production of albumin and other plasma proteins, cholesterol and bile acids. The liver is also the major organ which responsible for the metabolic bioactivation and detoxification of foreign chemicals. Although this organ, well endowed with defence systems, has the reserve capacity of withstanding to a limited degree chemically induced injury without impairment of normal physiological function, exposure to high doses can result in tissue damage leading to liver function failure. In this situation, changes in the levels of plasma and serum constituents are seen. Thus, plasma levels of albumin, total globulins, α_1-antitrypsin, ceruloplasmin, haptoglobin and transferrin are reduced. The increased activities in the serum of a number of cytosolic enzymes derived mainly from the liver are also seen following injury to the organ. The enzyme activities particularly affected are alanine aminotransferase and aspartate aminotransferases (ALT and AST respectively) and LDH. In situations where liver damage involves the development of cholestatic jaundice, serum alkaline phosphatase (ALP) and gamma-glutamyl transferase (GGT) activities are elevated. Liver function tests measuring bilirubin levels in serum and urine, urobiliogen in urine, and ALT, AST and ALP enzyme activities in serum have been used to distinguish between hepatic and cholestatic jaundice.

Kidney The kidneys and the renal system by the continuous excretion of excess water and metabolic waste products and by the selective reabsorption of electrolytes constitute the major organ for regulating the composition of water soluble constituents in the body. Other functions of the kidneys include gluconeogenesis (glucose synthesis), hormone production and secretion (renin and erythropoietin), and the metabolic activation of Vitamin D. When the renal clearance of water and solutes is obstructed either due to intrinsic kidney disease or as a consequence of chemical injury, or due to the obstruction of the urinary tract by renal tract stones, urine volume voided is reduced (oliguria) and plasma levels of urea and creatinine are markedly elevated. Increased urinary levels of plasma proteins, haemoglobin, myoglobin and immunoglobulins indicate renal tubular damage and/or interstitial disease. Heavy metals and some drugs are known to produce tubular damage.

Heart Damage to the myocardium leads to the leakage of a number of proteins and enzymes associated with heart and skeletal muscle into the circulation. The muscle derived components of particular interest are the troponins, a regulatory complex of proteins which lie against tropomyosin strands in muscles, and the enzymes, CK, AST and LDH. These proteins and enzymes have been found to exist as distinct isoform variants in heart muscles enabling their source to be identified. Thus, troponin T and troponin I isoforms are characteristic of heart muscle source, whereas troponin C exists in only one form and is distributed in all muscles. Raised plasma levels of troponin T have been found immediately following myocardial infarction, whereas troponin I is released into the circulation over a prolonged period following heart muscle damage, and is therefore considered to be a better indicator of heart attack. Isozymes of creatine kinase and lactate dehydrogenase derived from the heart have also been characterised and the measurement of the activities of CK(MB) and LDH(HBD) isoforms have been shown to reflect heart muscle damage.

Thyroid gland Thyroxine (T_4) and tri-iodothyronine (T_3) the two hormones, produced by the thyroid gland on stimulation by the pituitary derived TSH, are released into blood bound to plasma proteins. The concentration of T_4 in blood is about 70-fold greater than that of T_3. Changes in the blood levels of T_4, T_3 and TSH are reliable indicators of thyroid function. Hyperactivity of thyroid function is characterised by increased blood levels of T_4 and T_3 and decreased level of TSH. Conversely, low blood levels of T_4 and T_3 and a high level of TSH indicate hypothyroidism.

Pancreas Several disease conditions are known to adversely affect pancreatic function, including acute and chronic pancreatitis, cystic fibrosis, an inherited metabolic disease, and cancers of the pancreas. A number of chemicals have also been found to produce pancreatic damage. The presence of the exocrine enzymes, amylase and lipase in serum been found to be useful indicators of disordered pancreatic function. As both of these enzymes have relatively low molecular masses, they are cleared from the circulation by the kidneys and can be detected in the urine.

7.4.1 Hypothalamus-pituitary-adrenal axis

The inter-linked and interdependent action of these three tissues plays a pivotal role in controlling the synthesis and function of the cascade of hormones of the mammalian endocrine system. As mentioned in Section 7.4, the hypothalamus secretes several polypeptide regulatory factors into the blood supplying the anterior pituitary gland thereby triggering the production of a range of hormones responsible for the production of ultimate hormones by other target glands. Interruption of normal function in any of the various sectors of the endocrine system caused either by disease or by chemical toxicity has the predictable chain reaction effect downstream from the site of injury. Furthermore, this interruption in due course may also disrupt the regulatory up-stream feed-back mechanism. The measurement of circulating levels of marker polypeptides and hormones provides a useful indication of the primary site of damage to the endocrine system. Some of the hormonal markers of anterior pituitary dysfunction are prolactin, GH, ACTH, LH and FSH. Changes in the circulating levels of vasopressin and oxytocin indicate damage to the posterior pituitary gland. In the case of the adrenal gland, the markers in the serum indicative of dysfunction are cortisol, ACTH, aldosterone (the mineralocorticoid responsible for the reabsorption of sodium from the distal convoluted tubule of the kidney) and androgens.

Table 7.10 summarises the changes in various biochemical markers in body fluids described and reported in the literature to be indicative of damage to various organs and tissues. This list is by no means complete either in terms of the range of target organs affected or in terms of changes in biochemical parameters following tissue injury. The books recommended for further reading should help provide a fuller picture of changes reflecting dysfunction in other tissues.

It must be emphasised that the target organ shown and the specific intracellular organelle lesion indicated are the sites most sensitive to chemical injury at low doses of a chemical. Higher doses would inevitably overcome any protective mechanisms present in other organs resulting in generalised toxicity in the test species.

7.5 METHODOLOGIES – GENERAL

Many of the clinical biochemical methods routinely employed in chemical pathology laboratories for estimating proteins, activities of enzymes, levels of hormones and other substances

Table 7.10 Changes in biochemical markers in body fluid indicative of target organ toxicity

Target organ	Clinical chemistry markers
Liver disease	
Decrease in Plasma activity/ concentration of:	Albumin, Total Globulin, A1 Antitrypsin, Ceruloplasmin, Haptoglobulin, Transferrin
Increase in serum activity/ concentration of:	Aspartate aminotransferase, Alanine aminotransferase, Lactic Dehydrogenase, 5′ nucleotidase, Alkaline Phosphatase, Gamma Glutayml transferase
Kidney Disease	
Increase in Plasma concentration of:	Urea, Creatinine
Increase in Serum concentration of:	Normal plasma proteins, Haemoglobin, Myoglobin, Immunoglobulin, Glucose
Heart Disease	
Increase in Serum activity/ concentration of:	Creatine Kinase, Lactic Dehydrogenase, Asparate Aminotransferase, Troponin
Thyroid Gland	
Decrease in concentration of Thyroid Hormones in gland Hypoactivity and increase in Hyperactivity	[Thyroid Hormones] Thyroxine (T4), Tri-iodothyronine (T3), Thyrotropin (TSH)
Pancreatic Disease	
Increase in serum activity/ concentration of Amylase and Lipase	Increase in urine activity/ concentration of Amylase and Lipase
Hypothalamus-Pituitary-Adrenal axis	
Increase in serum. A range of endocrine protein markers	

present in biological fluids are standardised procedures approved by appropriate national and international professional bodies and in most cases the recommended analytical methods are automated. This section will therefore be confined to providing a general perspective of methods employed.

Electrophoretic techniques are used for separating various proteins present in serum and semi-quantified following staining with an appropriate dye to visualise the protein bands. More sensitive and specific methods involve the use of immunological techniques. Thus, blood levels of troponins T, C and I can be measured by specific enzyme-linked immunosorbent assay (ELISA) using monoclonal antibodies. Variations of methods based on these techniques have been found to have wider application in measuring not only proteins, including isoforms of the cytochrome P-450 proteins and isozymes of enzymes, but also hormone levels in body fluids and in tissues.

In the context of chemical toxicology, it is important to identify the chemical responsible for human toxicity. Biological monitoring is a well established technique for assessing intakes and uptakes of toxic elements following either occupational or environmental exposure. Recent analytical developments in atomic absorption spectrometry with electrothermal atomisation and of inductively coupled plasma-mass spectrometry allows the accurate measurement of all the stable inorganic elements in a small volume of blood. These techniques have been used for detecting human exposure to manganese, mercury and lead.

In the case of human exposure to dietary and environmental carcinogens, for example, aflatoxin, heterocyclic aromatic hydrocarbons, polycyclic aromatic hydrocarbons and aromatic amine, methods based on the measurement of DNA and protein adducts present in the blood and urine have been shown to provide reliable indicators in human population surveys. These methods have been extended to whole range of other environmental chemicals posing potential health risk to man.

A list of publications on the subject have been included in the books recommended for further reading.

7.6 SUMMARY AND CONCLUSION

This chapter attempts to provide a broad overview of the identity and location in organs and tissues of some of the important biochemical systems involved in maintaining normal physiological function in experimental animals and in man. This is reflected in well-defined limits of a number of biochemical markers present in biological fluids of healthy individuals. Following human exposure to a chemical many of these biochemical systems associated with organs and tissues mediate the metabolism, disposition and elimination of the chemical from the body. Metabolic processes result either in the detoxification of the chemical or to its bio-activation with the formation of toxic products. The latter situation can lead to the development in the target organ of a biochemical lesion, disturbance of normal physiological function and the manifestation of tissue injury. This results in changes in the levels of a number of biochemical markers originating from the affected organ in body fluids. Thus, the measurement of a range of representative biochemical constituents in body fluids, can provide a useful indication of organ toxicity in the intact animal. The main biochemical markers of diagnostic value in circulating blood are enzymes, proteins and hormones. A brief description of major con-stituents of mammalian biochemical systems and their relevance in chemical toxicology and in clinical chemistry follows.

Enzymes Enzymes are complex protein structures that act as biological catalysts mediating a wide range of trans-formation reactions. In the mammalian system, they are responsible for the metabolism of ingested dietary nutrients, such as, proteins, fats, carbohydrates and essential minerals and vitamins, for generating energy sources required for the efficient functioning of an organism and for the repair, replacement and growth of vital endogenous constituents in various organs and tissues in the body. The IUBMB has grouped the various enzymes into six main classes based on the general type of biotransformation reaction effected: (1) oxido-reductases; (2) hydrolases; (3) isomerases; (4) transferases; (5) lyases; and (6) ligases. Each of these classes are further divided into sub-classes based either on the substrate utilised (e.g. phospholipases) or a specific reaction mediated (e.g. glucuronyl transferases). Information on the enzyme systems and their intracellular location are given in the text.

The MFO enzyme system centred on the haemoprotein cytochrome P-450 and located intracellularly in the endoplasmic reticulum is mainly responsible for bioactivation and detoxification reactions effected on foreign chemicals. Cytochrome P-450 has been found to be composed of a number of isoforms of proteins, each with characteristic biocatalytic properties. The observed interindividual differences in the metabolism and toxicity of chemicals (polymorphism) is ascribable to variations in the composition of the isoforms of cytochrome P-450 present in the ER.

Damage inflicted in a target organ by a toxic chemical, leads to the leakage of "soluble" enzymes (i.e. not bound to intracelluar constituents), located in the cytoplasm, into the circulation and the estimation of enzyme activities in serum provides a useful indication of the target organ affected.

Proteins A variety of the proteins are present in plasma and many of these are synthesised in the liver. The main functions of the proteins in the circulation are to maintain colloid oncotic pressure, in the case of albumin, fulfil a carrier role (for example, albumin, ceruloplasmin, transferrin and thyroxine-binding globulin) and contribute to the body's immune defence system (e.g. the immunoglobulins). Changes in the circulating levels of specific proteins reflect morbidity and chemical toxicity. Thus, for example, increased circulating levels of the Troponins (-T and -I forms), derived from tropomyosin strands in muscles, are indicative of myocardial damage, and plasma level of ceruloplasmin, a copper containing protein, is reduced in Wilson's disease and in the nephrotic syndrome. Proteins derived from tumours in certain organs have been found in blood and the detection of these proteins may be indicative of the presence of the particular type of malignancy. Thus, for example, raised circulating levels of prostate specific antigen (PSA), a glycoprotein, may suggest prostate cancer and elevated levels of alpha fetoprotein (AFP) have been found in patients presenting with lumps in the testes. However, caution must be exercised in the interpretation of the findings as elevated levels of these proteins are not invariably reliable indicators of the presence of tumours, supporting evidence from other investigations is required to confirm diagnosis.

Hormones The hypothalamus-pituitary-adrenal axis plays a pivotal role in controlling the synthesis and supply of hormones required for regulating essential physiological functions in various organs in the body. Neurotransmitters stimulated by the central nervous system act on the hypothalamus triggering the release of a range of hypothalamic releasing hormones in the blood supply directed to the anterior pituitary gland. These stimuli acting on the anterior pituitary lead to a cascade of messengers to other organs, such as the thyroid, the adrenals, the kidneys and the reproductive systems involved in hormone production. Circulating blood is the main vehicle for the transport and supply of hormone-releasing factors and hormones required for the normal functioning of various organs and tissues. The measurement of plasma levels of these substances provides a valuable indicator of hormonal status in normal and diseased organs.

Analytical methods for the measurement of relevant biochemical markers in biological fluids, such as blood, urine and cerebro-spinal fluid, have not been included in this general review as standardised procedures are officially prescribed and should be referred to for details. Many of the methods are now automated and pre-packaged reagents available commercially. Considerable research has been directed to the development of specific methodologies for the biomonitoring of human populations for exposure to environmental chemicals. This has a useful preventative role in occupation and environmental medicine.

Chapter 8

Haematology

Haematology is the study of blood and of its disorders; it includes the blood forming organs (bone marrow). Blood can be considered to be a liquid organ and, together with blood forming tissues, is one of the largest in the body with a circulating blood volume of approximately 70 mL/kg bodyweight in humans. The ratio of blood volume to bodyweight is similar in the mammalian species commonly used in toxicology studies. Blood consists of the liquid phase or plasma, approximately 45% of the volume, and the formed elements, the red cells (erythrocytes), white cells (leucocytes) and platelets. The plasma contains a wide range of proteins, of which the largest quantity is albumin. Small amounts of electrolytes and other chemicals are also present. Chapter 7 deals with many of the changes that occur in the plasma.

The key role of the blood is the transport of nutrients and oxygen to all of the body and to transfer back excretory products, including carbon dioxide, to their sites of elimination. Minor, but essential chemicals, such as hormones are transported in the blood as are xenobiotics and their metabolites. The latter contributes to the distribution of the xenobiotic to various tissues, a factor essential in understanding tissue-specific toxicity.

The blood is contained within the arteries, arterioles, capillaries, venules, and veins as well as the sinuses of some tissues such as the blood-forming bone marrow and the spleen. The smaller vessels, particularly the capillaries, permeate all tissues in the body to allow the transport of nutrients and oxygen to all cells.

8.1 CYTOLOGY

A characteristic of mammals is relatively a high metabolic rate requiring a continuous relatively large supply of oxygen. The red cells are uniquely adapted for this mission. They constitute approximately 40% of the blood volume, depending on species, and impart the red colour to the blood due to the presence of the iron-containing pigment, haemoglobin. Under condition of high oxygen tension as in the lungs, haemoglobin binds oxygen and the circulation transports it to the tissues where it is released under the conditions of relatively low oxygen status.

The red cell is approximately 7 μm in diameter, a size greater than that of many capillaries. Hence, a key property of the erythrocyte is to be able to deform to reach all of the tissue cells. This deformability is achieved by being devoid of a nucleus (a characteristic of erythroid cells that is unique to mammals), and by the shape of the cell. The nucleus is expelled during the final cell division of the progenitor cell in the bone marrow. The red cells have a biconcave discoid shape that provides a large surface area to volume ratio com-

Table 8.1 The life cycle of red and white cells

Red cells	White cells
Stem cell	Stem cell
Erythroblast	Myeloblast
Normoblast	Promyelocyte
Reticulocyte	Myelocyte
Red blood corpuscle	Meta myelocytes
	Band cells
	Polymorphonuclear myelocyte

pared with the more normal near spherical shape of cells. Although this large ratio aids rapid gas exchange, it also allows the cell to deform to pass through narrow capillaries. The loss of this ability of the cells to deform and development of rigidity of the red-cell membrane, as part of the ageing process, cause them to be trapped when passing through small pores in, for example, the bone marrow or spleen. This is a key factor in assessing the age of the cell.

There are two main types of white cells: (1) the neutrophilic polymorphonuclear cell (neutrophil); and (2) the lymphocyte, although minor populations of others (eosinophilic, basophilic and monocytes) are present. The classification is based on their appearance and staining properties, especially of cytoplasmic granules, in microscopic preparations. The neutrophils cells have a lobulated nucleus and are involved in the phagocytosis of foreign materials including infective agents. They are able to migrate from the vessels as part of the inflammatory process. The other main group of white cells, the lymphocyte, is recognised by a large round nucleus, a small proportion of cytoplasm and a smaller size than the polymorphs. Lymphocytes are involved in the recognition of foreign proteins and the production, processing and distribution of antibodies. As such they are key to the immune process with numerous functional subpopulations but this is outside the range of this chapter (see Chapter 7).

The third formed element found in the blood is called platelets. They are smaller than erythrocytes. They are not complete cells but fragments of cytoplasm from the bone-marrow progenitor cell, the megakaryocyte. Platelets are central to the clotting mechanisms to avoid blood loss following injury.

8.2   HAEMATOLOGY AND TOXICOLOGY STUDIES

It is now realised that because of the central role of blood in promoting good health and homeostasis measurements of haematological indices has been a requirement in toxicity studies for many years, particularly those for regulatory purposes. A range of haematological measurement could be carried out on small species on the recommendation of regulatory authorities. When these requirements were first included, the range of measurements that could be carried out, especially using small species such as mouse rat and marmoset was limited by the relatively small volume of blood that could be collected and by the analytical method available. The sample sizes were not a limitation with the commonly used larger species such as the dog or larger monkey. With the improvements in the available technology a much wider range of measurements can now be made with the limited samples that can be collected from small animals.

In addition to being laborious and time consuming, the older manual and optical methods were subject to considerable variation. For example, enumerating red cells using visual counting by microscope and special counting-chamber slides examined relatively small numbers of cells and involved large dilution factors leading to inaccuracies in the counts. Since the data generated by the modern electronic equipment are based on analysis of large numbers of cells, they are less variable than those using the older methods. Because of these improvements, the information available to the toxicologist is reliable and provides a basis for understanding the pathogenesis of the effects encountered.

The haematology data generated during toxicology studies provide a picture of the status of the blood at one or a few time-points during the course of the study. It is common for these to be reported simply as increases or decreases relative to the untreated controls, usually only those that are statistically significant different. Further, the effect and no-effect doses are defined in relation to these differences. The cell numbers in the circulating blood at any time-point are a dynamic balance of the rate of their production, their survival in the circulation and the rate of destruction. A careful consideration "snapshots" of the static data and the relationships between the various measurements can allow them to be interpreted in terms of the dynamic process and this can be considered as the challenge of interpreting the results.

*In addition to the measurements made on the blood, findings from clinica and *post-mortem* observations, organ weights and histopathological findings can contribute to the interpretation of the haematological processes. Furthermore, holistic approach is capable of providing more information on the pathogenesis of the toxicological process than the simple identification of treatment-related differences from the normal.

8.2.1 Factors affecting quality

This section will consider some factors that could affect the quality of haematological data, the measurements that are generally made, the dynamic interpretation of the findings and some examples of results from toxicological tests with an interest in haematology.

Although it is relatively easy to acquire samples, reliable haematological information can only be obtained from high quality blood samples. They should be representative of the circulating blood, the volume must be adequate to carry out the measurements and it must be treated to prevent clotting. Ethylenediamine tetra-acetic acid (EDTA) is the usual anticoagulant and is the most effective for preventing clumping of the platelets allowing accurate counting. A separate sample taken into citrate will be required for measuring aspects of the clotting function. Commercial collecting tubes can be obtained. These are treated with the anticoagulants so that, if the correct volume of blood is added, the correct concentration of anticoagulant will be present.

The blood should be free flowing when collected. If there is stasis at the site of collection, haemoconcentration resulting in abnormally high counts is likely to occur. Collecting adequate samples from superficial vessels of large animals is relatively easy although, mechanical trauma, may develop accidentally (for example, if excessive vacuum develops when using syringes), and must be avoided to prevent rupture of red cells. A lack of such precautions could hide toxic effects since changes in cellular fragility can be a toxic response. Equally, the samples must be handled carefully when transferring from syringes to the sample tubes and when rotating the tubes to ensure solution of the anticoagulant. Bleeding may be difficult if the clotting mechanisms are altered by the test substance or if the cardiovascular condition is affected, perhaps leading to low blood pressure or collapse of the vessels. Using collecting equipment treated with anticoagulant can help to overcome such difficulties.

Obtaining adequate samples from small animals can be more difficult than from the larger species. In the rat, for example, blood can be collected from a superficial (usually tail) vessel, from the retro orbital sinus or from a major vessel such as the aorta or vena cava. The last method can provide relatively large samples but can only be carried out as part of a terminal procedure. As such it can be used only once and the animals will be under the influence of an anaesthetic. In skilled hands, the puncture of the retro-orbital sinus with a capillary tube can provide adequate samples but, again, anaesthesia is needed and the possibility of interference between the anaesthetic and the compound under investigation needs to be considered. Ethically, it is not possible to bleed on repeated occasions using this method. Blood can be collected from a tail vein either by a simple puncture or, preferably, using a syringe or cannula. These vessels collapse easily and, to maintain an adequate blood flow, frequently the environmental temperature is increased for a short period to dilate the vessels before collecting the sample.

If more than one sample is to be collected during a study, it is important that the same site of collection is used throughout to ensure that the data are comparable. For example, in a series of studies investigating the safety of food additives, the number of leucocytes in samples taken from the tail during the course of the study were higher than those in samples taken from the aorta at the end of the experiment. In one typical study the control leucocyte counts in males and females were $24.9 \times 10^3 \text{mm}^3$ and $20.2 \times 10^3 \text{mm}^3$ respectively in samples collected from the tail at week seven of the study. At 13 weeks using samples collected from the aorta the values were $7.0 \times 10^3 \text{mm}^3$ and $5.3 \times 10^3 \text{mm}^3$. This was not an effect of the age of the animals since the values ranged from $6.9 \times 10^3 \text{mm}^3$ to $7.8 \times 10^3 \text{mm}^3$ when the samples were collected at 2, 6 and 13 weeks from the aorta of subgroups of rats.

Animal welfare considerations and regulations strictly limit the volumes of blood and the frequency with which they are collected from various species. These factors must be taken into account when designing studies in order to gain the maximum information with the minimum of stress to the experimental subjects. Regulatory toxicity studies usually require that, at a minimum, haematology is examined at the end of the treatment period. In large-animal studies, involving relatively small numbers of experimental subjects, it is usual to conduct an examination before treatment, allowing the results after treatment with a xenobiotic to be compared with the base line for the individual animals as well as with untreated, control animals. If animal welfare considerations permit, useful information can be gained from early examinations and in studies of longer than 4 weeks duration, interim examinations can be helpful.

8.3 HISTORICAL DATA

It is important that each laboratory collects and tabulates control data to provide a historical database. This allows the experimental findings to be placed in context as an addition to the comparison with the study control data and any pre-treatment base-line information. This historical data has to be collected separately in relation to species, strain, sex and age of the animals. It can be used to ensure that the study controls are within the expected ranges as well as to put the experimental findings, particularly small deviations from the controls, into context. Nonetheless, such background data have to be used with care. Because of the chance of outliers in the populations, a simple comparison with the overall range is unlikely to be rewarding and may well serve to obscure subtle changes. A correct statistical use of the information to define the likely ranges can be very valuable. Also, this information can be monitored for any drifts in the data with time. These may be due to genetic drift in the animal populations or changes in husbandry practices. The drifts should not result from changes in the analytical techniques as since recognised standard samples should be included in the analyses. The experimental results are only accepted if the values with these results are within the acceptable limits. These samples are centrally standardised and provide both internal quality control and a form of comparison between studies in different laboratories.

The usual range of measurements that can be generated by modern instruments is shown in Table 8.2 although this will vary somewhat between laboratories and the equipment that is used. In all systems, the concentration of haemoglobin is measured. The numbers of formed elements, red cells, white cells and platelets are counted and sized. Depending on the system used, the formed elements are counted and their volumes measured based on conductivity changes due to displacement of the electrolyte diluent or by methods based

Table 8.2 Measurements commonly included in haematological examinations

Erythrocyte count	Platelet count
Haemoglobin concentration	Platelet crit (relative volume of platelets)
Packed cell volume (haematocrit)	Platelet distribution width
Mean cell volume	Total leukocyte count
Mean cell haemoglobin	Differential leukocyte count
Mean cell haemoglobin concentration	Reticulocyte count
Erythrocyte distribution width	Prothrombin time
Haemoglobin concentration width	Partial thromboplastin time

on flow cytometry. From these measurements, various other indices are calculated. These indices are measures of the population means for size and haemoglobin content of the erythrocytes and size of the platelets. Because modern instruments measure the volume of a large number of individual cells, it is possible to calculate not only average values but also the distribution of the size of the cell population.

It is possible to enumerate specific cell populations such as reticulocytes (newly formed red cells) and the different types of white cells with some of the current instruments. However, it is common to enumerate these populations by examining specially stained microscopic preparations. For demonstrating reticulocytes, a small sample of blood is incubated with a solution of methylene blue or brilliant cresyl blue and a spread made for microscopic examination. The different types of leucocytes are counted using a blood smear stained by the Giemsa method. Even when the subpopulations are counted by automated methods, the microscopic examination of a carefully prepared and Giemsa blood smear by an experienced haematologist can provide much useful information. It will reveal abnormally shaped cells that may be present in relatively small numbers and that, in most cases, would not affect the cell volumes or their distribution. Equally small populations of abnormal cells can be identified. The normal appearance of the red cell is a pale staining round cell with a smooth outline and an even paler centre due to the biconcave shape. The younger erythrocytes are darker staining with a blue tinge to the colour (polychromatic).

Absence of the pale centre suggests a loss of the discoidal shape, often associated with changes in membrane function. There may be also changes in the outline of the cells including irregularities or a spiky appearance. The proportion of the younger, polychromatic cells is likely to correlate with an increased number of reticulocytes indicating an increased cell production. A well-prepared blood smear allows differences in cell size to be defined, supporting the information generated from cell size distribution data. If the red cells or a subpopulation of them have a pale appearance, it suggests that they are deficient in haemoglobin.

The red cells may contain inclusions although these often require additional staining, such as for iron, to identify their nature. Nucleated erythrocytes, erythroblasts, are readily identified. Very small numbers of these nucleated erythrocytes can be found in normal animals, especially young individuals, but if they are increased in relation to the controls, these indicate a markedly increased production of red cells with release from the marrow earlier than usual. Small nuclei-like inclusions, micronuclei, may be seen. Frequently genotoxic (chromosome damaging) compounds cause these. They are usually a single chromosome or fragment not included in the nuclear membrane and not extruded during the final division of the progenitor cells.

As well as defining the proportions of the different types of leucocytes usually present in the circulation, the examination of a blood smear allows abnormal cell types to be identified. For example, cell types normally confined to the marrow may be present especially if the production is stimulated.

The number of the third formed element, platelets, is one index of the condition of the clotting mechanism but it is usual to include other indices of this mechanism in the basic range of measurements. The common indices included are pro-thrombin time and partial thromboplastin time using samples collected into trisodium citrate anticoagulant.

As well as the measurements described and commonly included in toxicity studies (Table 8.2), there are numerous other examinations that can be included. The investigations required will depend on the mechanism of toxicity being investigated but some examples are listed in Table 8.3.

If there is reason to expect a specific effect, from previous knowledge or chemical analogy, some of these might be included in the "routine" toxicity study. More commonly, however, they will form part of specific experiments to investigate mechanisms of toxicity.

Table 8.3 Examples of measurements that may be included
for the investigation of haematological effects

Differential bone-marrow count
Histology of marrow
Methaemoglobin concentration
Heinz bodies
Osmotic fragility
Reduced glutathione concentration
Erythrocyte deformability
Bone marrow colony forming ability

The detailed microscopic examination of a bone-marrow smear can yield information on effects, either suppression or stimulation of particular stages of the red (erythroid) and/or white (myeloid) cell production. A common approach is to collect marrow at *post-mortem* examination and prepare stained microscopic preparations but to examine them only if other data suggest an effect. Since these data are expressed as the proportions within the sample available, usually taken from the femur, they do not give a picture of the overall capacity of the marrow. For example, the proportion of the cells in the sample taken might be within normal ranges whilst the total cell population of the marrow is either greater or less than normal. To understand the capacity of the marrow, the proportions of the various types of cells must be combined with general views of the cellularity of the sample examined together with histological evidence of marrow hypoplasia or hyperplasia and the extent of extramedullary haemopoiesis in tissues such as the spleen or liver. For a complete diagnosis this evaluation must be considered together with the evidence from the peripheral blood. In the case of the erythrocyte, this would include the number of reticulocytes, polychromasia in the blood smear and the presence of nucleated cells.

In the leucocytes, a consideration of the extent of the lobulation of the nucleus polymorphs can give information of their production. Since the nucleus tends to be more lobular as the cell ages, a relatively greater lobulation would be expected if their production is inhibited. The reverse would be expected under conditions of increased production and forms of the cells normally confined to the marrow can appear in the circulation.

Methaemoglobin is a form of the pigment with the iron oxidised and incapable of carrying oxygen. Methaemoglobin together with Heinz bodies are caused by xenobiotics capable of causing oxidative changes. Both occur when the reducing capacity of the erythrocyte, mainly in the form of reduced glutathione is exceeded. Methaemoglobin is formed during the normal functioning of the red cells but they contain enzymatic systems for reducing it and to reduce glutathione. The activity of these systems declines with the age of the cells so that they become increasingly susceptible. In addition, there are genetic polymorphisms of some of the key enzymes involved in these processes. In particular, some human populations are deficient in glucose-6-phosphate dehydrogenase (G-6-PD), an enzyme involved in providing the energy for the reduction of glutathione and, hence, protecting the cell from oxidation. These populations are sensitive to the action of potentially oxidative drugs such as the aminoquinoline antimalarial drugs, for example, primaquine and dapsone. Because of the ability of the erythrocyte to reduce methaemoglobin, it should be measured as soon as possible after collecting the blood sample.

In conclusion, haematology is regularly included in toxicology studies and has long been a requirement of the guidelines for regulatory studies. Since blood and its ability to transport oxygen is vital to maintain the normal status and functioning of the body, it is important to demonstrate that it is not adversely affected by xenobiotics. The haematological status can contribute to an understanding of the general health of the animals involved in toxicity studies. The results obtained, however, are more than a series of measurements to be described in terms of increases or decreases compared with the normal. Rather, they are inter-related indices that, together with other, related observations from the study, can provide mechanistic explanations of toxic mechanisms.

Glossary

Absolute lethal concentration (LC_{100}) Lowest concentration of a substance in an environmental medium which kills 100% of test organisms or species under defined conditions. This value is dependent on the number of organisms used in its assessment.

Absolute lethal dose (LD_{100}) Lowest amount of a substance which kills 100% of test animals under defined conditions. This value is dependent on the number of organisms used in its assessment.

Absorbed dose (of a substance) Amount of a substance absorbed into an organism or into organs and tissues of interest.

Absorption (biological) Process of active or passive transport of a substance into an organism: in the case of a mammal or human being, this is usually through the lungs, gastrointestinal tract or skin.

Absorption (in colloid and surface chemistry)   Process whereby, when two phases are brought into contact, a particular component is transferred from one phase to the other.

Absorption (of radiation)   Phenomenon in which radiation transfers some or all of its energy to matter which it traverses.

Absorption coefficient (in biology)   Ratio of the absorbed amount (uptake) of a substance to the administered amount (intake): for exposure by way of the respiratory tract, the co-efficient is the ratio of the absorbed amount to the amount of the substance (usually particles) deposited (adsorbed) in the lungs.

Abuse (of drugs, substances, solvents etc.)   Improper use of drugs or other substances.

Acceptable daily intake (ADI)   Estimate of the amount of substance in food or drinking water, expressed on a body mass basis (usually mg/kg body weight), which can be ingested daily over a lifetime by humans without appreciable health risk. For calculation of the daily intake per person, a standard body mass of 60 kg is used. Acceptable daily intake is normally used for food additives (tolerable daily intake is used for contaminants).

Acceptable residue level of an antibiotic   Acceptable concentration of a residue which has been established for an antibiotic found in human or animal foods.

Acceptable risk   Probability of suffering disease or injury which is considered to be sufficiently small to be "negligible".

Accepted risk   Probability of suffering disease or injury which is accepted by an individual.

Accidental exposure   Unintended contact with a substance or change in the physical environment (including, for example, radiation) resulting from an accident.

Acclimatisation (biological)
1   Processes, including selection and adaptation, by which a population of micro-organisms develops the ability to degrade a substance, or develops a tolerance to it.

2   In animal tests – allowing an animal to adjust to its environment prior to undertaking a study.

Accumulation   Successive additions of a substance to a target organism, or organ, or to part of the environment, resulting in an increasing amount or concentration of the substance in the organism, organ or environment.

Acidosis   Pathological condition in which the hydrogen ion substance concentration of body fluids is above normal and hence the pH of blood falls below the reference interval.

Action level

1   Concentration of a substance in air, soil, water or other defined medium at which specified emergency counter-measures, such as the seizure and destruction of contaminated materials, evacuation of the local population or closing down the sources of pollution, are to be taken.

2   Concentration of a pollutant in air, soil, water or other defined medium at which some kind of preventive action (not necessarily of an emergency nature) is to be taken.

Acute effect   Effect of short duration and occurring rapidly (usually in the first 24 h or up to 14 d) following a single dose or short exposure to a substance or radiation.

Acute toxicity test   Experimental animal study to determine what adverse effects occur in a short time (usually up to 14 d) after a single dose of a substance or after multiple doses given in up to 24 h.

Adaptation

1   Change in an organism, in response to changing conditions of the environment (specifically chemical), which takes place without any irreversible disruptions of the given biological system and without exceeding normal (homeostatic) capacities of its response.

2   Process by which an organism stabilises its physiological condition after an environmental change.

Added risk   Difference between the incidence of an adverse effect in a treated group (or organisms or a group of exposed humans) and a control group (of the same organisms or the spontaneous incidence in humans).

Addiction   Surrender and devotion to the regular use of a medicinal or pleasurable substance for the sake of relief, comfort, stimulation, or exhilaration which it affords; often with craving when the drug is absent.

Additive effect   Consequence which follows exposure to two or more physico-chemical agents which act jointly but do not interact: commonly, the total effect is the simple sum of the effects of separate exposure to the agents under the same conditions. Substances of simple similar action may show dose or concentration addition.

Adduct   New chemical species AB, each molecular entity of which is formed by direct combination of two separate molecular entities A and B in such a way that there is no change in connectivity of atoms within their moieties A and B. Stoichiometries other than 1:1 are also possible. An intramolecular adduct can be formed when A and B are groups contained within the same molecular entity.

Adenocarcinoma   Malignant tumour originating in glandular epithelium or forming recognizable glandular structures.

Adenoma   Benign tumour occurring in glandular epithelium or forming recognisable glandular structures.

Adjuvant
   1   In pharmacology, a substance added to a drug to speed or increase the action of the main component.
   2   In immunology, a substance (such as aluminium hydroxide) or an organism (such as bovine tuberculosis bacillus) which increases the response to antigen.

Administration (of a substance)   Application of a known amount of a substance to an organism in a reproducible manner and by a defined route.

Adrenergic   Sympathomimetic.

Adsorption Enrichment (positive adsorption, or briefly adsorption) of one or more components in an interfacial layer.

Adverse effect Change in morphology, physiology, growth, development or life span of an organism which results in impairment of functional capacity or impairment of capacity to compensate for additional stress or increase in susceptibility to the harmful effects of other environmental influences.

Adverse event Occurrence which causes an adverse effect.

Aerobic Requiring molecular oxygen.

Aerodynamic diameter (of a particle) Diameter of a spherical particle of unit density which has the same settling velocity in air as the particle in question.

Aerosol Dispersion of liquid or solid material in a gas.

Aetiology

1 Science dealing with the cause or origin of disease.

2 Individuals, the cause or origin of disease.

After-effect of a poison Ability of a poison to produce a change in an organism after cessation of contact.

Age sensitivity Quantitative and qualitative age dependence of an effect.

Agonist Substance which binds to cell receptors normally responding to naturally occurring substances and which produces a response of its own.

Air pollution Presence of substances in the atmosphere resulting wither from human activity or natural processes, in sufficient concentration, for a sufficient time and under circumstance such as to interfere with comfort, health or welfare of persons or to harm the environment.

Air pollution control system

1 Network of organisations which monitor air pollution.

2 Group of measures or processes used to minimise or prevent air pollution.

Algicide Substance intended to kill algae.

Alkylating agent Substance which introduces an alkyl substituent into a compound.

Allergy   Symptoms or signs occurring in sensitised individuals following exposure to a previously encountered substance (allergen) which would otherwise not cause such symptoms or signs in non-sensitised individuals. The most common forms of allergy are rhinitis, urticaria, asthma, and contact dermatitis.

Anabolism   Biochemical processes by which smaller molecules are joined to make larger molecules.

Anaemia   Condition in which there is a reduction in the number of red blood cells or amount of haemoglobin per unit volume of blood below the reference interval for a similar individual of the species under consideration, often causing pallor and fatigue.

Anaerobe   Organism which does not need molecular oxygen for life. Obligate (strict) anaerobes grow only in the absence of oxygen. Facultative anaerobes can grow either in the presence or in the absence of molecular oxygen.

Anaerobic   Not requiring molecular oxygen.

Analgesic   Substance which relieves pain, without causing loss of consciousness.

Analogue metabolism   Process by which a normally non-biodegradable compound is biodegraded in the presence of a structurally similar compound which can induce the necessary enzymes.

Analytic study (in epidemiology)   Hypothesis-testing method of investigating the association between a given disease or health state or other dependent variable and possible causative factors in an analytic study, individuals in the study population are classified according to absence which may influence disease occurrence. Attributes may include age, race, sex, other disease(s), genetic, biochemical and physiological characteristics, economic status, occupation, residence and various aspects of the environment or personal behaviour. Three types of analytic study are: (1) cross-sectional (prevalence); (2) cohort (prospective); and (3) case control (retrospective).

Anaphylaxis Severe allergic reaction occurring in a person or animal exposed to an antigen or hapten to which they have previously been sensitised.

Anaplasia Loss of normal cell differentiation, a feature characteristic of most malignancies.

Aneuploid Cell or organism with missing or extra chromosomes or parts of chromosomes.

Anoxia Strictly total absence of oxygen but sometimes used to mean decreased oxygen supply in tissues.

Antagonism Combined effect of two or more factors, which is smaller than the solid effect of any one of those factors. In bioassays, the term may be used when a specified response is produced by exposure to either of two factors but not by exposure to both together.

Antagonist

1 Substance that reverses or reduces the effect induced by an agonist.

2 Substance that attaches to and blocks cell receptors that normally bind naturally occurring substances.

Anthelmint(h)ic Substance intended to kill parasitic intestinal worms, such as helminths.

Anthracosis (coal miners' pneumoconiosis). Form of pneumoconiosis caused by accumulation of carbon deposits in the lungs due to inhalation of smoke or coal dust.

Anthropogenic Caused by or influenced by human activities.

Antibiotic Substance produced by, and obtained from, certain living cells (especially bacteria, yeasts and moulds), or an equivalent synthetic substance, which is biostatic or biocidal at low concentrations to some other form of life, especially pathogenic or noxious organisms.

Antibody Protein molecule produced by the immune system (an immunoglobulin molecule) which can bind specifically to the molecule (antigen or hapten) which induced its synthesis.

Anticoagulant Substance which prevents clotting.

Antidote Substance capable of specifically counteracting or reducing the effect of a potentially toxic substance in an organism by a relatively specific chemical or pharmacological action.

Antigen   Substance or a structural part of a substance which causes the immune system to produce specific antibody or specific cells and which combines with specific binding sites (epitopes) on the antibody or cells.

Antimetabolite   Substance, structurally similar to a metabolite, which competes with it or replaces it and so prevents or reduces its normal utilisation.

Antimycotic   Substance used to kill a fungus or to inhibit its growth.

Antipyretic   Substance which relieves or reduces fever.

Antiresistant   Substance used as an additive to a pesticide formulation in order to reduce the resistance of insects to the pesticide.

Antiserum   Serum containing antibodies to a particular antigen wither because of immunisation or after an infectious disease.

Aphasia   Loss or impairment of the power of speech or writing, or of the ability to understand written or spoken language or signs, due to a brain injury or disease.

Aplasia   Lack of development of an organ or tissue, or of the cellular products from an organ or tissue.

Apoptosis   Physiological process of programmed tissue death (and disintegration) associated with normal development in animals.

Argyria   Pathological condition characterised by grey-bluish or black pigmentation of tissues (such as skin, retina, mucous membranes, internal organs) caused by the accumulation of metallic silver, due to reduction of a silver compound which has entered the organism during (prolonged) administration or exposure.

Arrhythmia   Any variation from the normal rhythm or the heartbeat.

Artefact   Finding or product of experimental or observational techniques that is not properly associated with the system being studied.

Arteriosclerosis Hardening and thickening of the wall of the arteries.

Arthritis Inflammation of a joint, usually accompanied by pain and often by changes structure.

Asbestosis Form of pneumoconiosis caused by inhalation of asbestos fibres.

Asphyxia Condition resulting from insufficient intake of oxygen: symptoms include breathing difficulty, impairment of senses, and in extreme, convulsions, unconsciousness and death.

Assay

1   Process of quantitative or qualitative analysis of a component of a sample.

2   Results of a quantitative or qualitative analysis of a component of a sample.

Assessment of exposure See NT biological assessment of exposure.

Asthenia Weakness; lack or loss of strength.

Asthma Chronic respiratory disease characterised by bronchoconstriction, excessive mucus secretion and oedema of the pulmonary alveoli, resulting in difficulty in breathing out, wheezing, and cough.

Ataxia Unsteady or irregular manner of walking or movement caused by loss or failure of muscular co-ordination.

Atherosclerosis Pathological condition in which there is thickening, hardening, and loss of elasticity of the walls of blood vessels, characterised by a variable combination of changes of the innermost layer consisting of local accumulation of lipids, complex carbohydrates, blood and blood components, fibrous tissue and calcium deposits. In addition, the outer layer becomes thickened and there is fatty degeneration on the middle layer.

Autophagosome Membrane-bound body (secondary lysosome) in which parts of the cell are digested.

Autopsy *Post-mortem* examination of the organs and body tissue to determine cause of death or pathological condition.

Bactericide Substance intended to kill bacteria.

Base pairing Linking of the complementary pair of polynucleotide chains of nucleic acids by means of hydrogen bonds between complementary purine and pyrimidine bases, adenine with thymine or uracil, cytosine with guanine.

Bias Deviation of results or inferences from the truth, or processes leading to such deviation. Any trend in the collection, analysis, interpretation, publication or review data which can lead to conclusions which are systematically different from the truth. Among the ways in which deviation from the truth can occur are the following:

1   Systematic (one-sided) variation of measurements from the true values.

2   Variation of statistical summary measures (means, rates, measures of association etc.) from their true values as a result of systematic variation of measurements, other flaws in data collection, or flaws in study design or analysis.

3   Deviation of inferences from the truth as a result of flaws in study design, data collection, or the analysis or interpretation of results.

4   A tendency of procedures (in study design, data collection, analysis, interpretation review or publication) to yield results or conclusions which depart from the truth.

5   Prejudice leading to the conscious or unconscious selection of study procedures which depart from the truth in a particular direction, or to one-sidedness in the interpretation of results.

Bioactivation Any metabolic conversion of a xenobiotic to a more toxic derivative.

Bioavailability

1   Extent to which a substance to which the body is exposed (by ingestion, inhalation, injection, or skin contact) reaches the systemic circulation, and the rate at which this occurs.

2   Pharmacokinetic term relating systemic exposure from extravascular exposure (ev) to that following intravenous exposure (iv) by the equation:

$$F = AUC_{ev} * D_{iv}/AUC_{iv} * D_{ev}$$

where F is the bioavailability, AUC_{ev} and AUC_{iv} are the areas under the plasma concentration time curve following extravascular and intravenous administration and D_{ev} and D_{iv} are the administered extravascular and intravenous doses.

Biochemical mechanism   Reaction or series of reactions, usually enzyme-catalysed, associated with a specific physiological event in a living organism.

Biocid/e n., -al *adj.*   Substance intended to kill living organisms.

Bioconcentration   Process leading to a higher concentration of a substance in an organism than in environmental media to which it is exposed.

Biodegradation   Breakdown of a substance catalysed by enzymes *in vitro* or *in vivo*. This may be characterised for purposes of hazard assessment as:

1   Primary: Alteration of the chemical structure of a substance resulting in loss of a specific property of that substance.

2   Environmentally acceptable: Biodegradation to such an extent as to remove undesirable properties of the compound. This often corresponds to primary biodegradation but it depends on the circumstances under which the products are discharged into the environment.

3   Ultimate: Complete breakdown of a compound to either fully oxidised or reduce simple molecules (such as carbon dioxide/methane, nitrate/ammonium, and water.

It should be noted that the produces of biodegradation can be more harmful than the substance degraded.

Bio-elimination   Removal, usually from the aqueous phase, of a test substance in the presence of living organisms by biological processes supplemented by physico-chemical reaction.

Biological assessment of exposure

1   Assessment of exposure to a substance by the analysis of specimens taken in the environment such as foodstuffs, plants, animals, biological material in air or water samples, or biological material from exposed subjects. When human samples are analysed, they are usually urine and blood; other possible samples includes expire air, faeces, saliva, bile, hair and biopsy or autopsy material. When other organisms are being considered, the whole organism may be analysed as well as selected tissues such as fat in pigs or birds. In these samples, the content(s) of the substance(s) or metabolite(s) is determined and, on this basis, the exposure level (concentration in the air, absorbed amount of the substance) or the probability of health impairment due to exposure are derived.

2   Biochemical changes in the components of an organism, such as changes in enzyme activity or in the excretion of metabolic intermediates, can also be used for this purpose if they show a relationship to the exposure.

Biological monitoring   Continuous or repeated measurement of potentially toxic substances of their metabolites or biochemical effects in tissues, secreta, excreta, expired air or any combination of these in order to evaluate occupational or environmental exposure and health risk by comparison with appropriate reference values based on knowledge of the probable relationship between ambient exposure and resultant adverse health effects.

Biota   All living organisms as a totality.

Biotransformation   Any chemical conversion of substances that is mediated by living organisms or enzyme preparation derived therefrom.

Body burden Total amount of substance of a chemical present in an organism at a given time.

Brady- Prefix meaning slow as in bradycardia or bradypnoea.

Bradycardia Abnormal slowness of the heart.

Builder Material which enhances or maintains the cleaning efficiency of a surfactant, in a detergent, principally by inactivating water hardness; complex phosphates (especially sodium tripolyphosphate, i.e. pentasodium triphosphate), sodium carbonate and sodium silicate are the builders most commonly used.

Calcification Process in which organic tissue becomes hardened by deposition of calcium salts within its substance.

Cancer Disease resulting from the development of a malignancy.

Carboxyhaemoglobin Compound which is formed between carbon monoxide and haemoglobin in the blood of animals and which is incapable of transporting oxygen.

Case control study A study which starts with the identification of persons with the disease (or other outcome variable) of interest, and a suitable control (comparison, reference) group of persons without the disease. The relationship of an attribute to the disease is examined by comparing the diseased and non-diseased with regard to how frequently the attribute is present or, of quantitative, the levels of the attribute, in the two groups.

Catabolism

1   Reactions involving the oxidation of organic substrates to provide chemically available energy (for example ATP) and to generate metabolic intermediates.

2   Generally, process of breakdown of complex molecules into simpler ones, often providing biologically available energy.

Ceiling value (CV) The US term in occupational exposure indicating the airborne concentration of a potentially toxic substance which should never be exceeded in a worker's breathing zone.

Cell line Defined unique population of cells obtained by culture from a primary implant through numerous generations.

Cell-mediated hypersensitivity State in which an individual reacts with allergic effects caused by the reaction of antigen-specific T-lymphocytes following exposure to a certain substance (allergen) after having been exposed previously to the same substance or chemical group.

Cell-mediated immunity Immune response mediated by antigen-specific T-lymphocytes.

Cell strain Cells having specific properties or markers derived from a primary culture or cell line.

Chemical conversion Change from one state or chemical structure to another.

Chemical safety Practical certainty that there will be no exposure of organisms to toxic amounts of any substance or group of substances: this implies attaining an acceptably low risk of exposure to potentially toxic substances.

Chemical species Set of chemically identical atomic or molecular structural units of solid array or of chemically identical molecular entities that can explore the same set of molecular energy levels on the time scale of the experiment. For example, two conformational isomers may interconvert sufficiently slowly to be detectable by separate nuclear magnetic resonance spectra and hence be considered to be separate chemical species on a time scale governed by the radio frequency of the spectrometer used. On the other hand, in a slow chemical reaction the same mixture of conformers may behave as single chemical species, i.e. there is a virtually complete equilibrium population of the total set of molecular energy levels belonging to the two conformers. Except where context requires otherwise, the term is taken to refer to a set of molecular entities containing isotopes in their natural abundance. The wording of the definition given intended to embrace both cases such as graphite, sodium chloride, or a surface oxide, where the basic structured units are not capable of a separate existence as well as those cases where they are.

Chromosomal aberration Abnormality of chromosome number or structure.

Chromosome Self-replicating structure consisting of DNA complexed with various proteins and involved in the storage and transmission of genetic information; the physical structure that contains the genes.

Chronic effect Consequence which develops slowly and has a long-lasting course (often but not always irreversible).

Chronic toxicity

1   Adverse effects following chronic exposure.

2   Effects which persist over a long period of time whether or not they occur immediately upon exposure or are delayed.

Chronic toxicity test Study in which organisms are observed during the greater part of the life span and in which exposure to the test agent takes place over the whole observation time or a substantial part thereof.

Circulation of substances in the environment Movement of xenobiotic substance in the environment with air flow, river current, soil, water, etc.

Cirrhosis

1   Liver disease defined by histological examination and characterised by increased fibrous tissue, abnormal physiological changes such as loss of functional liver capacity and increased resistance to blood flow through the liver (portal hypertension).

2   Interstitial fibrosis of an organ.

Clearance

1   Volume of blood or plasma or mass of an organ effectively cleared of a substance by elimination (metabolism and excretion) in a given time interval: clearance is expressed in units of volume or mass per unit of time. Total clearance for a component is the

sum of the clearances of each eliminating organ or tissue for the component.

2   In pulmonary toxicology, clearance refers specifically to removal of any inhaled substance which deposits on the lining surface of the lung: lung clearance is expressed in volume or mass of lung cleared per unit time.

3   In renal toxicology, clearance refers to the quantification of the removal of a substance by the kidneys by the processes of filtration and secretion: clearance is calculated by relating the rate of renal excretion to the plasma concentration.

Clon/e., -al *adj.*

1   Population of genetically identical cells or organisms having a common ancestor.

2   To produce such a population.

3   Recombinant DNA molecules all carrying the same inserted sequence.

Cocarcinogen   Chemical, physical or biological factor which intensifies the effect of a carcinogen.

Cohort   Component of the population born during a particular period and identified by period of birth so that its characteristics (such as causes of death and numbers still living) can be ascertained as it enters successive time and age periods. The term "cohort" has broadened to describe any designated group of persons followed or traced over a period of time, as in the term cohort study (prospective study).

Cohort analysis   Tabulation and analysis of morbidity or mortality rates in relationship to the ages of a specific group of people (cohort), identified by their birth period, and followed as they pass through different ages during part or all of their life span. In certain circumstances such as studies of migrant populations, cohort analysis may be performed according to duration of residence in a country rather than year of birth, in order to relate health or mortality experience to duration of exposure.

Cohort study Method of epidemiological study in which subsets of a defined population can be identified who are, have been, or in the future may be exposed or not exposed, or exposed in different degrees, to a factor or factors hypothesised to influence the probability of occurrence of a given disease or other outcome. Alternative terms for such a study – follow-up, longitudinal, and prospective study – describe an essential feature of the method, observation of the population for a sufficient number of person-years to generate reliable incidence or mortality rates in the population subsets. This generally means studying a large population, study for a prolonged period (years, or both).

Compensation Adaptation of an organism to changing conditions of the environment (especially chemical) is accompanied by the emergence of stresses in biochemical system which exceed the limits of normal (homeostatic) mechanisms. Compensation is a temporary concealed pathology which later on can be manifested in the form of explicit pathological changes (de-compensation).

Concentration–effect curve Graph of the relation between exposure concentration and the magnitude of the resultant biological change.

Confounding

1 Situation in which the effects of two processes are not distinguishable from one another: the distortion of the apparent effect of an exposure on risk brought about by the association of other factors which can influence the outcome.

2 Relationship between the effects of two or more causal factors as observed in a set of data, such that it is not logically possible to separate the contribution which any single causal factor has made to an effect.

3 Situation in which a measure of the effect of an exposure on risk is distorted because of the association of exposure with other factor(s) which influence the outcome under study.

Conjunctiva Mucous membrane which covers the eyeball and lines the under-surface of the eyelid.

Contaminant

1 Minor impurity present in a substance.

2 Extraneous material inadvertently added to a sample prior to or during chemical biological analysis.

3 In some contexts, as in relation to gas cleaning equipment, used as a synonym for "pollutant", especially on a small scale.

4 Unintended component in food that may pose a hazard to the consumer.

Control group Selected group, identified as a rule before a study is done, which comprises humans, animals, or other species who do not have the disease, intervention, procedure or whatever is being studied, but in all other respects is as nearly identical to the test group as possible.

Control, matched Control (individual or group or case) selected to be similar to a study individual or group, or case, in specific characteristics: some commonly used matching variables are age, sex, race and socio-economic status.

Corrosive Causing a surface-destructive effect on contact; in toxicology, this normally means causing visible destruction of the skin, eyes, or the lining of the respiratory tract or the gastrointestinal tract.

Criterion Validated set of data used as a basis for judgement.

Critical concentration (for a cell or organ) Concentration of a potentially toxic substance at which undesirable (or adverse) functional changes, reversible or irreversible, occur in the cell or organ.

Cross-sectional study (of disease prevalence and associations) Study which examines the relationship between diseases (or other health-related characteristics) and other variables of interest as they exist in a defined population at one particular time. Disease prevalence rather than incidence is normally recorded in a cross-sectional study and the temporal sequence of cause and effect cannot necessarily be determined.

Cumulative effect Overall adverse change which occurs when repeated doses of a harmful substance or radiation have biological consequences which are mutually enhancing.

Cyanosis Bluish coloration, especially of the skin and mucous membranes and fingernail beds, caused by abnormally large amounts of reduced haemoglobin in the blood vessels as a result of deficient oxygenation.

Cytochrome Haemoprotein whose characteristic mode of action involves transfer of reducing equivalents associated with a reversible change in oxidation state of the haemprosthetic group; strictly, the cytochrome P-450 family are not cytochromes but haemthiolate proteins.

Cytochrome P-420 Inactive derivative of cytochrome P-450 found in microsomal preparations.

Cytochrome P-448 Obsolete term for cytochrome P-450 I, A1 and A2, one of the major families of the cytochromes P-450 haemoproteins. During the mono-oxygenation of certain substances, often a detoxification process, these iso-enzymes may produce intermediates which initiate mutations, chemical carcinogenesis, immunotoxic reactions and other forms of chemical toxicity.

Cytochrome P-450 Haemoproteins which form the major part of the enzymes concerned with the mono-oxygenation of many endogenous and exogenous substrates. The term includes a large number of iso-enzymes which are coded for a superfamily of genes. Endogenous substrates of these enzymes include cholesterol, steroid hormones and the eicosenoids; the exogenous substrates are xenobiotics. Strictly, the cytochrome P-450 family are not cytochromes but are haemthiolate proteins.

Death rate Estimate of the proportion of a population which dies during a specified period. The numerator is the number of persons dying during the period; the denominator is the size of the population, usually estimated as the mid-year population. The death rate in a population is generally calculated by the formula: (10^n number of deaths during s specified period)/ (Number of persons at risk of dying during the period). This rate is an estimate of the person-time death rate, the death rate per 10^n persons-year usually $n = 3$. If the rate is low, it is also a good estimate of the cumulative death rate. This rate is also called the crude death rate.

Decontamination Process of rendering harmless (by neutralisation, elimination, removal etc.) a potentially toxic substance in the natural environment, laboratory areas, the workplace, other indoor areas, clothes, food, water sewage etc.

Defoliant Substance used for removal of leaves by its toxic action on living plants.

Dehydrogenase Enzyme which catalyses oxidation of compounds by removing hydrogen.

Delayed effect Consequence occurring after a latent period following the end of exposure to a toxic substance or other harmful environmental factor.

Denaturation

1   Addition of methanol or acetone to alcohol to make it unfit for drinking.

2   Change in molecular structure of proteins so that they cannot function normally, often caused by splitting of hydrogen bonds following exposure to reactive substances or heat.

Deoxyribonucleic acid (DNA) Constituent of chromosomes which stores the hereditary information of an organism in the form of a sequence of purine and pyrimidine bases: this information relates to the synthesis of proteins and hence it is a determinant of all physical and functional activities of the cell, and consequently of the whole organism.

Dependence

1 A psychic craving for a drug or other substance which may or may not be accompanied by a physical dependency.

2 Reliance on a drug or other substance to maintain health.

Deposition

1 Process by which a substance arrives at a particular organ or tissue site, for example, the deposition of particles on the ciliated epithelium of the bronchial airways.

2 Process by which a substance sediments out of the atmosphere or water and settles in a certain place.

Dermal Pertaining to the skin.

Dermal irritation Skin reaction resulting from a single or multiple exposure to a physical or chemical entity at the same site, characterised by the presence of inflammation; it may result in cell death.

Desensitisation Suppression of sensitivity of an organism to an allergen to which the organism has been exposed previously.

Desiccant

1 Drying agent.

2 In agriculture, a substance used for drying up plants and facilitating their mechanical harvesting.

Diploid Chromosome state in which the chromosomes are present in homologous pairs. Normal human somatic (non-reproductive) cells are diploid (they have 46 chromosomes) whereas reproductive cells, with 34 chromosomes, are haploid.

Discontinuous effect See SN intermittent effect.

Distribution

1 Dispersal of a substance and its derivatives throughout the natural environment.

2 Dispersal of a substance within an organism, including metabolism, storage and excretion.

3 Final location of a substance within an organism after dispersal.

Diuresis   Excretion of urine, especially in excess.

Diuretic   Agent which increases urine production.

Dosage   Dose expressed as a function of the organism being dosed and time, for example, mg/(kg body weight)/day. See dose.

Dose   Total amount of substance administered to, taken or absorbed by an organism. Absolute lethal dose, cumulative medial lethal dose, lethal dose, maximum tolerable dose, maximum tolerated dose, median effective dose, median lethal dose, median narcotic dose, minimum lethal dose, non-effective dose, organ dose, threshold dose, toxic dose.

Dose–effect curve   Graph of the relation between dose and the magnitude of the biological change produced measured in appropriate units.

Dose–effect relationship   Association between dose and the magnitude of a continuously graded effect, either in an individual or in a population or in experimental animals.

Dose-related effect   Situation in which the magnitude of a biological change is proportional to the dose.

Dose–response curve   Graph of the relation between dose and the proportion of individuals in a population responding with an all-or-none effect.

Dose–response relationship   Association between dose and the incidence of a defined biological effect in an exposed population.

Draize test   Evaluation of materials for their potential to cause dermal or ocular irritation and corrosion following local exposure; generally using the rabbit model (almost exclusively the New Zealand White) although other animal species have been used.

Drug   Any substance which when absorbed into a living organism may modify one or more of its functions. The term is generally accepted for a substance taken for a therapeutic purpose, but is also commonly used for abused substances.

Duplicate (replicate) samples (in chemistry) Two (or multiple) samples taken under the same or comparable conditions.

Dysarthria Imperfect articulation of speech due to neuro-muscular damage.

Dysplasia Abnormal development of an organ or tissue identified by morphological examination.

Dyspnoea Difficult or laboured breathing.

Ecology Branch of biology which studies the interactions between living organisms and all factors (including other organisms) in their environment: such interactions encompass environmental factors which determine the distributions of living organisms.

Ecosystem Grouping of organisms (micro-organisms, plants, animals) interacting together, with and through their physical and chemical environments, to form a functional entity.

Ecotoxicology Study of the toxic effects of chemical and physical agents on all living organisms, especially on populations and communities within defined ecosystems; it includes transfer pathways of these agents and their interactions with the environment.

Ecoparasiticide Substance intended to kill parasites living on the exterior of the host.

Eczema Acute or chronic skin inflammation with erythema, papules, vesicles, pustules, scales, crusts or scabs, alone or in combination of varied aetiology.

Effective concentration (EC) Concentration of a substance that causes a defined magnitude of response in a given system: EC_{50} is the median concentration that causes 50% of maximal response.

Effective dose (ED) Dose of a substance that causes a defined magnitude of response in a given system: ED_{50} is the median dose that causes 50% of maximal response.

Embryo

1   Stage in the developing mammal at which the characteristic organs and organ systems are being formed: for humans, this involves the stages of development from the second to the eighth week (inclusive post conception).

2   In birds, the stage of development from the fertilisation of the ovum up to hatching.

3   In plants, the stage of development within the seed.

Embryotoxicity

1   Production by a substance of toxic effects in progeny in the first period of pregnancy between conception and foetal stage.

2   Any toxic effect on the conceptus as a result of prenatal exposure during the embryonic stages of development: these effects may include malformations and variations, malfunctions, altered growth, prenatal death and altered postnatal function.

Endemic   Present in a community or among a group of people; said of a disease prevailing continually in a region.

Endocrine   Pertaining to hormones or to the glands that secrete hormones directly into the bloodstream.

Endoplasmic reticulum (ER)   Intracellular complex of membranes in which proteins and lipids, as well as molecules for export, are synthesised and in which the biotransformation reactions of the mono-oxygenase enzyme systems occur: may be isolated as microsomes following cell fractionation procedures.

Endothelial   Pertaining to the layer of flat cells lining the inner surface of blood and lymphatic vessels, and the surface lining of serous and synovial membranes.

Environment   Aggregate, at a given moment, of all external conditions and influences to which a system under study is subjected.

Environmental damage   Adverse effects to the natural environment.

Environmental exposure level (EEL) Level (concentration or amount or a time integral of either) of a substance to which an organism or other component of the environment is exposed in its natural surroundings.

Environmental health Human welfare and its influence by the environment, including technical and administrative measures for improving the human environment from a point of view.

Environmental health criteria documents Critical publications of IPCS containing reviews of methodologies and existing knowledge – expressed, if possible, in quantitative terms – of selected substances (or groups of substances), on identifiable, immediate, and long-term effects on human health and welfare.

Environmental hygiene Practical control measures used to improve the basic environmental conditions affecting human health, for example clean water supply, human and animal waste disposal, protection of food from biological contamination, and housing conditions, all of which are concerned with the quality of the human environment.

Environmental impact assessment (EIA) Appraisal of the possible environmental consequences of a past, ongoing, or planned action, resulting in the production of an environmental impact statement or "finding of no significant impact (FONSI)".

Enzootic Present in a community or among a group of animals; said of a disease prevailing continually in a region.

Epidemiology Study of the distribution and determinants of health-related states or events in populations and the application of this study to control of health problems.

Epigastric Pertaining to the upper-middle region of the abdomen.

Epithelioma Any tumour derived from epithelium.

Erythema Redness of the skin produced by congestion of the capillaries.

Eschar   Slough or dry scab on an area of skin.

Estimated daily intake (EDI)   Prediction of the daily intake of a residue of a potentially harmful agent based on the most realistic estimation of the residue levels in food and the best available food consumption data for a specific population: residue levels are estimated by taking into account known used of the agent, the range of contaminated commodities, the proportion of a commodity treated, and the quantity of home-grown or imported commodities.

Estimated exposure concentration (EEC)   Measured or calculated amount or mass concentration of a substance to which an organism is likely to be exposed, considering exposure by all sources and routes.

Estimated exposure dose (EED)   Measured or calculated dose of a substance to which an organism is likely to be exposed, considering exposure by all sources and routes.

Estimated maximum daily intake (EMDI)   Prediction of the maximum daily intake of a residue of a potentially harmful agent based on assumptions of average food consumption per person and maximum residues in the edible portion of a commodity, corrected for the reduction or increase in residues resulting from preparation, cooking, or commercial processing. The EMDI is expressed in mg residue per person.

Eutrophic   Describes a body of water with a high concentration of nutrient salts and a high or excessive rate of biological production.

Excretion   Discharge or elimination of an absorbed or endogenous substance, or of a waste product, and/or their metabolites, through some tissue of the body and its appearance in urine, faeces, or other products normally leaving the body. Excretion of chemical compounds from the body occurs mainly through the kidney and the gut. Volatile compounds may be largely eliminated by exhalation. Excretion by perspiration and through hair and nails may also occur. Excretion by the gastrointestinal tract may take place by various routes such as the bile, the shedding of intestinal cells and transport through the intestinal mucosa.

Exposure

1 Concentration, amount or intensity of a particular physical or chemical agent or environmental agent that reaches the target population, organism, organ, tissue or cell, usually expressed in numerical terms of substance concentration, duration, and frequency (for chemical agents and micro-organisms) or intensity (for physical agents such as radiation).

2 Process by which a substance becomes available for absorption by the target population, organism, organ, tissue or cell, by any route.

Exposure assessment Process of measuring or estimating concentration (or intensity), duration and frequency of exposures to an agent present in the environment or, of estimating hypothetical exposures, that might arise from the release of a substance, or radionuclide, into the environment.

Exposure limit General term defining an administrative substance concentration or intensity of exposure that should not be exceeded.

Exposure–response relationship See RT dose–response relationship.

Extrapolation Calculation, based on quantitative observations in exposed test species *in vitro* test systems, of predicted dose–effect and dose–response relationships for a substance in humans and other biota including interspecies extrapolations and extrapolation to susceptible groups of individuals: the term may also be used for qualitative information applied to species or conditions that are different from the ones which the original investigations were carried out.

Fetus (often incorrectly foetus) Young mammal within the uterus of the mother from the visible completion of characteristic organogenesis until birth: in humans, this period is usually defined as from the third month after fertilisation until birth (prior to this, the young mammal is referred to as an embryo).

Fixed dose procedure Acute toxicity test in which a substance is tested initially at a small number (three or four) predefined doses to identify which produces evident toxicity without lethality: the test may be repeated at one or more higher or lower defined discriminating doses to satisfy the criteria.

Food additives Any substance not normally consumed as a food by itself and not normally used as a typical ingredient of the food, whether or not it has nutritive value, the intentional addition of which to food for a technological (including organoleptic) purpose in the manufacture, processing, preparation, treatment, packing, packaging, transport or holding of such food results, or may by reasonably expected to result (directly or indirectly) in it or its byproducts becoming a component of or otherwise affecting the characteristics of such foods. The term does not include "contaminants" or substances added to food for maintaining or improving nutritional qualities.

Food allergy Hypersensitivity reaction to substances in the diet to which an individual has previously been sensitised.

Food chain Sequence of transfer of matter and energy in the form of food from organism to organism in ascending or descending trophic levels.

Food intolerance Physiologically based reproducible, unpleasant (adverse) reaction of a specific food or food ingredient that is not immunologically based.

Gamete Reproductive cell (either sperm or egg) containing a haploid set of chromosomes.

Gametocide Substance intended to kill gametes.

Gavage Administration of materials directly into the stomach by oesophageal intubation.

Gene Structurally a basic unit of hereditary material; an ordered sequence of nuclei bases that encodes one polypeptide chain (following transcription to mRNA).

Gene amplification Production of extra copies of a chromosomal sequence found either as intra- or extra-chromosomal DNA; with respect to a plasmid, it refers to the increase in the number of plasmid copies per cell induced by a specific treatment of transformed cells.

Genome Complete set of chromosomal and extrachromosomal genes of an organism, a cell, and organelle, or a virus; complete DNA component of an organism.

Genotoxicity Ability to cause damage to genetic material. Such damage may be mutagenic and/or carcinogenic.

Germ-free animal Animal grown under sterile conditions in the period of post-natal development; such animals are usually obtained by Caesarean operation and kept in special sterile boxes in which there are no viable microorganisms (sterile air, food and water are supplied).

Gnotobiont See SN gnotobiote.

Gnotobiot/e n., -ic *adj.* Specially reared laboratory animal whose microflora and microfauna are specifically known in their entirety.

Good laboratory practice (GLP) principles Fundamental rules incorporated in the national regulation concerned with the process of effective organisation and the conditions under which laboratory studies are properly planned, performed, monitored, recorded and reported.

Good manufacturing practice (GMP) principles Fundamental rules incorporated in national regulations concerned with the process of effective organisation of production and ensuring standards of defined quality at all staged of production, distribution and marketing; minimisation of waste and its proper disposal are part of this process.

Granuloma A tumour-like growth made up of M.E.F. M = macrophages; E = epithelial cells; F = fibroblasts and other cells.

Guinea-pig maximisation test (Magnusson and Kligman test)   Widely used skin test for screening possible contact allergens: considered to be a useful method to identify likely moderate and strong sensitisers in humans.

Haematemesis   Vomiting of blood.

Haematoma   Localised accumulation of blood, usually clotted, in an organ, space, or tissue, due to a failure of the wall of a blood vessel.

Haematuria   Presence of blood in the urine.

Haemolysis   Release of haemoglobin from erythrocytes, and its appearance in the plasma.

Haemosiderin   Iron-containing pigment that is formed for haemoglobin released during the disintegration of red blood cells and that accumulates in individuals who have ingested excess iron.

Half-life (half-time) (t1/2)   Time in which the concentration of a substance will be reduced by half, assuming a first order elimination process or radioactive decay.

Haploid (monoploid)   State in which a cell contains only one set of chromosomes.

Hapten   Low-molecular-weight molecule that contains an antigenic determinant (epitope) that may bind to a specific antibody but which is not itself antigenic unless complexed with an antigenic carrier such as a protein or cell; once bound it can cause the sensitisation of lymphocytes, possible leading to allergy or cell-mediated hypersensitivity.

Harmful substance   Substance that, following contact with an organism can cause ill health or adverse effects either at the time of exposure or later in the life of the present and future generations.

Hazard   Set of inherent properties of a substance, mixture of substances or a process involving substances that, under production, usage or disposal conditions, make it capable of causing adverse effects to organisms or the environment, depending on the degree of exposure; in other words, it is a source of danger.

Hazard assessment Determination of factors, controlling the likely effects of a hazard such as the dose–effect and dose–response relationships, variations in target susceptibility, and mechanism of toxicity.

Hazard evaluation Establishment of a qualitative or quantitative relationship between hazard and benefit, involving the complex process of determining the significance of the identified hazard and balancing this against identifiable benefit: this may subsequently be developed into a risk evaluation.

Hazard identification Determination of substances of concern, their adverse effects, target populations, and conditions of exposure, taking into account toxicity data and knowledge of effects on human health, other organisms and their environment.

Hazard quotient (HQ) Ration of toxicant exposure (estimated or measured) to a reference value regarded as corresponding to a threshold of toxicity: if the total hazard quotient from all toxicant to a target exceeds unity, the combination of toxicants may produce (will produce under assumptions of additivity) an adverse effect.

Hazardous production factor Production factor the effect of which on a worker under certain conditions results in injury or some impairment of health.

Health surveillance Periodic medico-physiological examinations of exposed workers with the objective of protecting health and preventing occupationally related disease.

Healthy worker effect Epidemiological phenomenon observed initially in studies of occupational diseases: workers usually exhibit lower overall disease and death rates than the general population, due to the fact that the old, severely ill and disabled are ordinarily excluded from employment. Death rates in the general population may be inappropriate for comparison, if this effect is not taken into account.

Homology   Degree of identity existing between the nucleotide sequences of two DNA molecules but not complementary DNA or RNA molecules; 70% homology means that on the average 70 out of every 100 nucleotides are identical in a given sequence. The same term is used in comparing the amino acid sequences of related proteins.

Hormesis   Stimulatory effect of small doses of a potentially toxic substance that is inhibitory in larger doses.

Hormone   Substance formed in one organ or part of the body and carried in the blood to another organ or part where it selectively alters functional activity.

Human ecology   Interrelationship between humans and the entire environment – physical, biological, socio-economic, and cultural, including the interrelationships between individual humans or groups of humans and other human groups or group of other species.

Hypertension   Persistently high blood pressure in the arteries or in a circuit, for example, pulmonary hypertension or hepatic portal hypertension.

Hypertrophy   Excessive growth in bulk of a tissue or organ through increase in size but not in number of the constituent cells.

Hypoxia

1   Abnormally low oxygen content or tension.

2   Deficiency of oxygen in the inspired air, in blood or in tissues, short of anoxia.

Idiosyncrasy   Genetically based unusually high sensitivity of an organism to that of certain substances.

Immission   Environmental concentration of a pollutant resulting from a combination of emissions and dispersals (often synonymous with exposure).

Immune complex   Product of an antigen–antibody reaction that may also contain components of the complement system.

Incidence   Number of occurrences of illness commencing, or of persons falling ill, during a given period in specific population: usually expressed as a rate, the denominator being the average number of persons in the specified population during a defined period or the estimated number of persons at the mid-point of that period. The basic distinction between "incidence" and "prevalence" is that whereas incidence refers only to new cases, prevalence refers to all cases, irrespective of whether they are new or old. When the terms incidence and prevalence are used, it should be stated clearly whether the data represent the numbers of instances of the disease recorded or the numbers of persons ill.

Incidence rate Measure of the frequency with which new events occur in a population. Value obtained by dividing the number of new events that occur in a defined period, sometimes expressed as person-time.

Induction period Time from the onset of exposure to the appearance of signs of disease.

Inhibitory dose (ID) Dose of a substance that causes a defined inhibition of a given system: ID_{50} is the median dose that causes 50% inhibition.

Initiator

1   Agent that induces a change in a chromosome or gene that leads to the induction of tumours after a second agent, called a promoter is administered to the tissue.

2   Substance that starts a chain reaction; an initiator is consumed in a reaction, contrast to a catalyst.

Intermittent effect Biological change that comes and goes at intervals.

Interspecies dose conversion Process of extrapolating from the doses of one animal species to another, for example, from rodent dose to human equivalent.

Interstitial pneumonia Chronic form of pneumonia involving increase of the interstitial tissue and decrease of the functional lung tissue.

Intestinal reabsorption Absorption further down the intestinal tract of a substance or substances that have been absorbed before and subsequently excreted into the intestinal tract usually through the bile.

Ionising radiation   Any radiation consisting of directly or indirectly ionising particles or a mixture of both or photons with energy higher than the energy of photons of ultraviolet light or a mixture of both such particles and photons.

Irreversible alteration   Change from normal structure or function that persists or progresses after cessation of exposure of the organism.

Irritant

1   *n.*, Substance that causes inflammation following immediate, prolonged or repeated contact with skin, mucous membrane, or other biological material. A substance capable of causing inflammation on first contact is called a primary irritant.

2   *adj.*, Causing inflammation following immediate, prolonged or repeated contact with skin, mucous membrane or other tissues.

Jaundice   Pathological condition characterised by deposition of bile pigment in the gut and mucous membranes, including the conjunctivae, resulting in yellow appearance of a patient or animal.

Joint effect   Simultaneous or successive effect of factors of diverse types (chemical, physical, and biological) on an organism.

Lachrymator   See lacrimator.

Lacrimator   Substance that irritates the eyes and causes the production of tears or increases the flow of tears.

Latent period   Delay between exposure to a disease-causing agent and the appearance and manifestations of the disease: also defined as the period from disease initiation to disease detection.

Lesion

1   Area of pathologically altered tissue.

2   Injury or wound.

3   Infected patch of skin.

Lethal   Deadly; fatal; causing death.

Lethal synthesis   Metabolic formation of a highly toxic compound from one that is relatively non-toxic (bioactivation), often leading to death of affected cells.

Leukaemia   Progressive, malignant disease of the blood-forming organs, characterised by distorted proliferation and development of leucocytes and their precursors in the bone marrow and blood.

Limit test   Acute toxicity test in which, if no ill-effects occur at a pre-selected maximum dose, no further testing at greater exposure levels is required.

Limit value (LV)   Limit concentration at or below which Member States of the European Community must set their environmental quality standard and emission standard for a particular substance according to Community Directives.

Limited evidence   According to the US environmental protection agency's (EPA) guidelines for Carcinogen Risk Assessment, "limited evidence" is a collection of facts and accepted scientific inference that suggests that an agent may be causing an effect, but this suggestion is not strong enough to be considered established fact.

Linearised multi-stage model   Sequence of steps in which (a) a multi-stage model is fitted to tumour incidence data; (b) the maximum linear term consistent with the data is calculated; (c) the low-dose slope of the dose–response function is equated to the coefficient of the maximum linear term; and (d) the resulting slope is then equated to the upper bound of potency.

Liposome   Originally a lipid droplet in the ER of a fatty liver. Now applied to an artificially formed lipid droplet, small enough to form a relatively stable suspension in aqueous media and with potential use in drug deliver.

Logit transformation   Mathematical transformation that relates response to a stated dose or concentration of a toxicant to the response in the absence of the toxicant by the formula:

$$\text{Logit} = 1\, g[B/(B_0 - B)]$$

where B is the response to the stated dose or concentration and B_0 is the response in the absence of the toxicant. Plotting the logit function against the logarithm of base 10 of the dose or concentration usually gives a linear relationship.

Lowest-observed-adverse-effect-level (LOAEL) Lowest concentration or amount of a substance, found by experiment or observation, which causes an adverse alteration of morphology, functional capacity, growth, development, or life span of a target organism distinguishable from normal (control) organisms of the same species and strain under defined conditions of exposure.

Lowest-observed-effect-level (LOEL) Lowest concentration or amount of a substance, found by experiment or observation, that causes any alteration in morphology, functional capacity, growth, development, or life span of target organisms distinguishable from normal (control) organisms of the same species and strain under the same defined conditions of exposure.

Lysosome Membrane-bound cytoplasmic organelle containing hydrolytic enzymes.

Morphages Large (10–20 mm diameter) amoeboid and phagocytic cell found in many tissues, especially in areas of inflammation; macrophages are derived from blood monocytes and play an important role in host defence mechanisms.

Magnusson and Kligman test See SN guinea-pig maximisation test.

Mainstream smoke (tobacco smoking) Smoke that is inhaled.

Malignant

1   Tending to become progressively worse and to result in death if not treated.

2   In cancer, cells showing both uncontrolled growth and a tendency to invade and destroy other tissues.

Margin of exposure (MOE), margin of safety (MOS)   Ration of the no-observed adverse-effect level (NOAEL) to the theoretical or estimated exposure dose (EED) or concentration (EEC).

Mass mean diameter   Diameter of a particle with a mass equal to the mean mass of the particles in a population.

Material safety data sheet (MSDS)   Compilation of information required under the USOSHA Hazard Communication Standard on the identity of hazardous substances, health and physical hazards, exposure limits, and precautions.

Maximum contaminant level (MCL)   Under the Safe Drinking Water Act (USA), primary MCL is a regulatory concentration for drinking water which takes into account both adverse effects (including sensitive populations) and technological feasibility (including natural background levels): secondary MCL is a regulatory concentration based on "welfare", such as taste and staining, rather than health, but also takes into account technical feasibility. MCL Goals (MCLG) under the Safe Drinking Water Act do not consider feasibility and are zero for all human and animal carcinogens.

Maximum exposure limit (MEL)   Occupational exposure limit legally defined in GB under COSHH as the maximum concentration of an airborne substance, averaged over a reference period, to which employees may be exposed by inhalation under any circumstances, and set on the advice of the HSC Advisory Committee on Toxic Substances.

Maximum permissible daily dose   Maximum daily dose of substance whose penetration into a human body during a lifetime will not cause diseases or health hazards that can be detected by current investigation methods and will not adversely affect future generations.

Maximum permissible level (MPL)   Level, usually a combination of time and concentration, beyond which any exposure of humans to a chemical or physical agent in their immediate environment is unsafe.

Maximum residue limit (MRL) for pesticide residues   Maximum contents of a pesticide residue (expressed as mg/kg fresh weight) recommended by the Codex Alimentarius Commission to be legally permitted in or on food commodities and animal feeds. Maximum residue limits are based on data obtained following good agricultural practice and foods derived from commodities that comply with the respective MRL's are intended to be toxicologically acceptable.

Maximum residue limit (MRL) for veterinary drugs   Maximum contents of a drug residue (expressed as mg/kg or ug/kg fresh weight) recommended by the Codex Alimentarius Commission to be legally permitted or recognised as acceptable in or on food commodities and animal feeds. The MRL is based on the type and amount of residue considered to be without any toxicological hazard for human health as expressed by the acceptable daily intake (ADI) or on the basis of a temporary ADI that uses and additional uncertainty factor. It also takes into account other relevant public health risks as well as food technological aspects.

Maximum tolerated dose (MTD)   High dose used in chronic toxicity testing that is expected on the basis of an adequate subchronic study to produce limited toxicity when administered for the duration of the test period. It should not induce: (a) overt toxicity, for example, appreciable death of cells or organ dysfunction; or (b) toxic manifestations that are predicted materially to reduce the life span of the animals except as the result of neoplastic development; or (c) 10% or greater retardation of body weight gain as compared with control animals. In some studies, toxicity that could interfere with a carcinogenic effect is specifically excluded from consideration.

Median effective concentration (EC$_{50}$) Statistically derived concentration of a substance in an environmental medium expected to produce a certain effect in 50% of test organisms in a given population under a defined set of conditions.

Median effective dose (ED$_{50}$) Statistically derived dose of a chemical or physical agent (radiation) expected to produce a certain effect in 50% of test organisms in a given population or to produce a half-maximal effect in a biological system under a defined set of conditions.

Median lethal concentration (LC$_{50}$) Statistically derived concentration of a substance in an environmental medium expected to kill 50% of organisms in a given population under a defined set of conditions.

Median lethal dose (LD$_{50}$) Statistically derived dose of a chemical or physical agent (radiation) expected to kill 50% of organisms in a given population under a defined set of conditions.

Median lethal time (TL$_{50}$) Statistically derived average time interval during which 50% of a given population may be expected to die following acute administration of a chemical or physical agent (radiation) at a given concentration under a defined set of conditions.

Median narcotic concentration (NC$_{50}$) Statistically derived concentration of a substance in an environmental medium expected to cause narcotic conditions in 50% of a given population under a defined set of conditions.

Median narcotic dose (ND$_{50}$) Statistically derived dose of a substance expected to cause narcosis in 50% of test animals under a defined set of conditions.

Mesothelioma Malignant tumour of the mesothelium of the pleura, pericardium or peritoneum, that may be caused by exposure to asbestos fibres and some other fibres.

Metaplasia   Abnormal transformation of an adult, fully differentiated tissues of one kind into a differentiated tissue of another kind.

Metastasis

1   Movement of bacteria or body cells, especially cancer cells, from one part of the body to another, resulting in change in location of a disease or of its symptoms from one part of the body to another.

2   Growth of pathogenic micro-organisms or of abnormal cells distant from their origin in the body.

Minimum lethal dose (LD$_{min}$)   Lowest amount of a substance that, when introduced into the body, may cause death to individual species of test animals under a defined set of conditions.

Mitochondri/on (*pl-a*)   Eukaryote cytoplasmic organelle that is bounded by an outer membrane and an inner membrane; the inner membrane has folds called cristae that are the centre of ATP synthesis in oxidative phosphorylation in the animal cell and supplement ATP synthesis by the chloroplasts in photosynthetic cells. The mitochondrial matrix within the inner membrane contains ribosomes, many oxidative enzymes, and a circular DNA molecule that carries the genetic information for a number of these enzymes.

Mitosis   Process by which a cell nucleus divides into two daughter nuclei, each having the same genetic complement as the parent cell: nuclear division is usually followed by cell division.

Mixed function oxidase   See SN mono-oxygenase.

Modifying factor (MF)   As used by USEPA, uncertainty factor that is greater than zero and less than, or equal to 10; the magnitude of the factor depends upon the professional assessment of scientific uncertainties of a study or database not explicitly treated with the standard uncertainty factors (for example the completeness of the overall database and the number of animals tested); the default value for the factor is 1.

Mono-oxygenase Enzyme that catalyses reactions between an organic compound and molecular oxygen in which one atom of the oxygen molecule is incorporated into organic compound and one atom is reduced to water; involved in the metabolism of natural and foreign compounds giving both unreactive products and products of reduced or increased toxicity from that of the parent compound: such enzymes are the main catalysts of phase 1 reactions in the metabolism of xenobiotics by the endoplasmic reticulum or by preparations of microsomes.

Multigeneration study

1　Toxicity test in which two to three generations of the test organism are exposed to the substance being assessed.

2　Toxicity in which only one generation is exposed and effects on subsequent generations are assessed.

Murine Of or belonging to the family of rats and mice *(Muridae)*.

Mutation Any relatively stable heritable change in genetic material that may be a chemical transformation of an individual gene (gene or point mutation, altering its function, or a rearrangement, gain or loss of part of a chromosome, that may be microscopically visible (chromosomal mutation); mutation can be either germinal and inherited by subsequent generations, or somatic and passed through cell lineage by cell division.

Natural occurrence Presence of a substance in nature, as distinct from presence resulting from inputs from human activities. The contamination of the natural environment by some man-made compounds may be so widespread that it is practically impossible to get access to biota with a truly natural level; only "normal" levels can be measured, those which are usually prevalent in places where there is no obvious local contamination.

Neoplas/ia, -m   New and abnormal formation of tissue as a tumour or growth by cell proliferation that is faster than normal and continues after the initial stimulus (I) that initiated the proliferation has ceased.

Nephritis   Inflammation of the kidney, leading to kidney failure, usually accompanied by proteinuria, haematuria, oedema and hypertension.

Nephrotoxic   Chemically harmful to the cells of the kidney.

Neuron(e)   Nerve cell, the morphological and functional unit of the central and peripheral nervous systems.

No-effect level (NEL)   Maximum dose (of a substance) that produces no detectable changes under defined conditions of exposure. At present, this term tends to be substituted by no-observed-adverse-effect-level (NOAEL) or no-observed-effect-level (NOEL).

No-observed-adverse-effect-level (NOAEL)   Greatest concentration or amount of a substance, found by experiment or observation, which causes no detectable adverse alteration of morphology, functional capacity, growth, development, or life span of the target organism under defined conditions of exposure.

Oliguria   Excretion of a diminished amount of urine in relation to fluid intake.

Oncogenesis   Production or causation of tumours.

Operon   Complete unit of gene expression and regulation, including structural genes, regulator gene(s) and control elements in DNA recognised by regulator gene product(s).

Organ dose   Amount of a substance or physical agent (radiation) absorbed by an organ.

Osteoporosis   Significant decrease in bone mass with increased porosity and increased tendency to fracture.

Ovicide   Substance intended to kill eggs.

Parasympathomimetic   Producing effects resembling those caused by stimulating the parasympathetic nervous system; also called cholinomimetic.

Parenteral dosage Method of introducing substances into an organism avoiding gastrointestinal tract (subcutaneously, intravenously, intramuscularly etc.).

Passive smoking Inhalation of sidestream smoke by people who do not smoke themselves.

Percutaneous Through the skin following application on the skin.

Perinatal Relating to the period shortly before and after birth; from the 20th to the 29th week of gestation to 1–4 weeks after birth.

Peroxisome Organelle, similar to a lysosome, characterised by its content of catalase (EC1.11.1.6), peroxidase (EC 1.11.1.7) and other oxidative enzymes.

Phagocytosis Engulfing and digestion of micro-organisms, other cells and foreign particles by cells such as phagocytes.

Pharmaceuticals Drugs, medical products, medicines, or medicaments.

Pharmacodynamics Process of interaction of pharmacologically active substances with target sites, and the biochemical and physiological consequences leading to therapeutic or adverse effects.

Phase 1 reaction (of biotransformation) Enzymic modification of a substance by oxidation, reduction, hydrolysis, hydration, dehydrochlorination or other reactions catalysed by enzymes of the cytosol, of the endoplasmic reticulum (microsomal enzymes or of other cell organelles).

Phase 2 reaction (of biotransformation) Binding of a substance, or its metabolites from a phase 1 reaction, with endogenous molecules (conjugation), making more water-soluble derivatives that may be excreted in the urine or bile.

Phase 3 reaction (of biotransformation) Further metabolism of conjugated metabolites produced by phase 2 reactions: it may result in the production of toxic derivatives.

Phenotype The observable structural and functional characteristics of an organism determined by its genotype and modulated by its environment.

Photo-irritation   Inflammation of the skin caused exposure to light, especially that due to metabolites formed in the skin by photolysis.

Photophobia   Abnormal visual intolerance of light.

Photosensitisation   Allergic reaction due to a metabolite formed by the influence of light.

Pleura   Lining of the lung.

Ploidy   Term indicating the number of sets of chromosomes present in an organism.

Pneumoconiosis   Usually fibrosis of the lungs that develops owing to (prolonged) inhalation of inorganic or organic dusts.

Cause-specific types of pneumoconiosis:

1   Anthracosis – from coal dust.
2   Asbestosis – from asbestos dust.
3   Byssinosis – from cotton dust.
4   Siderosis – from iron dust.
5   Silicosis – from silica dust
6   Stannosis – from tin dust.

Point mutation   Reaction that changes a single base pair in DNA.

Poison   Substance that, taken into or formed within the organism, impairs the health of the organism may kill it.

Porphyria   Disturbance of porphyrin metabolism characterised by increased formation, accumulation, and excretion of porphyrins and their precursors.

Potency   Expression of chemical or medicinal activity of a substance as compared to a given or implied standard or reference.

Potentiation   Dependent action in which a substance or physical agent at a concentration or dose that does not itself have an adverse effect enhances the harm done by another substance or physical agent.

Practical certainty (of safety)   Numerically specified low risk of exposure to a potentially toxic substance (for example, 1 in 10^6) or socially acceptable low risk of adverse effects from such an exposure applied to decision making in regard to chemical safety.

Prevalence Number of instances of existing cases of a given disease or other condition in a given population at a designated time; sometimes used to mean prevalence rate. When used without qualification, the term usually refers to the situation at a specified point in time (point prevalence).

Procarcinogen Substance that has to be metabolised before it can induce malignant tumours.

Prokaryote Unicellular organism, characterised by the absence of a membrane-enclosed nucleus. Prokaryotes include bacteria, blue-green algae and mycoplasmas.

Promoter (in oncology) Agent that induces cancer when administered to an animal or human being who has been exposed to a cancer initiator.

Prophage Latent state of a phage genome in a lysogenic bacterium.

Proportional mortality rate (ratio) (PMR) Number of deaths from a given cause in a specified time period, per 100 or per 1000 total deaths in the same time period: can give rise to misleading conclusions if used to compare mortality experience of populations with different causes of death.

Pyrexia Condition in which the temperature of a human being or mammal is above normal.

Quality assurance All those planned and systemic actions necessary to provide adequate confidence that a product or service will satisfy given requirements for quality.

Quality control
1 Operational techniques and activities that are used to fulfil requirements for quality.
2 In toxicology, procedures incorporated in experimental protocols to reduce the possibility of error, especially human error: this is a requirement of good laboratory practice.

Quantitative structure–activity relationship (QSAR) Quantitative association between the physico-chemical properties of a substance and/or the properties of its molecular substructures and its biological properties including its toxicity.

Rate difference (RD) Absolute difference between two rates, for example, the difference in incidence rate between a population group exposed to a causal factor and a population group not exposed to the factor: in comparisons of exposed and unexposed groups, the term "excess rate" may be used as a synonym for rate difference.

Receptor High affinity binding site for a particular toxicant.

Reference dose Term used for an estimate (with uncertainty spanning perhaps an order of magnitude) of a daily exposure to the human population (including sensitive subgroups) that is likely to be without appreciable risk of deleterious effects during a lifetime.

Relative risk

1   Ratio of the risk of disease or death among the exposed to that among the unexposed.

2   Ratio of the cumulative incidence rate in the exposed to the cumulative incidence rate in the unexposed; the cumulative incidence ratio.

Replication

1   Duplicated or repeated performance of an experiment under similar (controlled) conditions to reduce the error to a minimum, and to estimate the variations and thus obtain a more precise result; each determination, including the first is called a replicate.

2   Process whereby the genetic material is duplicated.

Reproducibility Closeness of agreement between test results obtained under reproducibility conditions.

Reproductive toxicant Substance or preparation that produces non-heritable harmful effects on the progeny and/or an impairment of male and female reproductive function on capacity.

Reserve capacity Physiological or biochemical capacity that may be available to maintain homeostasis when the body or an organism is exposed to an environmental change.

Response

1   Proportion of an exposed population with a defined effect or the proportion of a group of individuals

that demonstrate a defined effect in a given time at a given dose rate.

2   Reaction of an organism or part of an organism (such as a muscle) to a stimulus.

Retention

1   Holding back within the body or within an organ, tissue or cell of matter that is normally eliminated.

2   Holding in memory of what has been learned for later use as recall, recognition or relearning.

3   Amount of a substance that is left from the total absorbed after a certain time.

Reverse transcription   Process by which an RNA molecule is used as a template to make a single-stranded DNA copy.

Ribonucleic acid (RNA)   Linear, usually single stranded, polymer or ribonucleotides, each containing the sugar ribose in association with a phosphate group and one of 4 nitrogenous bases: adenine, guanine, cytosine, or uracil; it encodes the information for the sequence of amino-acids in proteins synthesised using it as a template.

Risk

1   Possibility that a harmful event (death, injury or loss) arising from exposure to a chemical or physical agent may occur under specific conditions.

2   Expected frequency of occurrence of a harmful event (death, injury or loss) arising from exposure to a chemical or physical agent under specific conditions.

Risk assessment   Identification and quantification of the risk resulting from a specific use or occurrence of a chemical or physical agent, taking into account possible harmful effects on individual people or society of using the chemical or physical agent in the amount and manner proposed and all the possible routes of exposure, quantification ideally requires the establishment of dose–effect and dose–response relationships in likely target individuals and populations.

Risk characterisation Outcome of hazard identification and risk estimation applied to a specific use of a substance or occurrence of an environmental health hazard: the assessment requires quantitative data on the exposure of organisms or people at risk in the specific situation. The end product is a quantitative statement about the proportion of organisms or people affected in a target population.

Risk estimation Assessment, with or without mathematical modelling, of the probability and nature of effects of exposure to a substance based on quantification of dose–effect and dose–response relationships for that substance and the population(s) and environmental components likely to be exposed and on assessment of the levels of potential exposure of people, organisms and environment at risk.

Risk management Decision-making process involving considerations of political, social, economic, and engineering factors with relevant risk assessments relating to a potential hazard so as to develop, analyse, and compare regulatory options and to select the optimal regulatory response for safety from that hazard. Essentially risk management is the combination of three steps: (1) risk-evaluation; (2) emission and exposure control; (3) risk monitoring.

Risk marker Attribute that is associated with an increased probability of occurrence of a disease or other specified outcome and that can be used as an indicator of this increased risk; not necessarily a causal or pathogenic factor.

Risk monitoring Process of following up the decisions and actions within risk management in order to check whether the aims of reduced exposure and risk are achieved.

Risk perception Subjective perception of the gravity or importance of the risk based on a person's knowledge of different risks and the moral, economic, and political judgement of their implications.

Sample

1   In statistics, a group of individuals often taken at random from a population for research purposes.

2   One or more items taken from a population or a process and intended to provide information on the population or process.

3   Portion of material selected from a larger quantity in some manner chosen so that the portion is representative of the whole.

Secondary metabolite   Product of biochemical processes other than the normal metabolic pathways, mostly produced in micro-organisms or plants after the phase of active growth and under conditions of nutrient deficiency.

Sensitivity (of a screening test)   Extent (usually expressed as a percentage) to which a method gives results that are free from false negatives; the fewer the false negatives, the greater the sensitivity. Quantitatively, sensitivity is the proportion of truly diseased persons in the screened population who is identified as diseased by the screening test.

Sensitisation   Immune process whereby individual become hypersensitive to substances, pollen, dandruff, or other agents that make them develop a potentially harmful allergy when they are subsequently exposed to the sensitising material (allergen).

Side-effect   Action of a drug other than that desired for beneficial pharmacological effect.

Sidestream smoke   Cloud of small particles and gases that is given off from the end of a burning tobacco product (cigarette, pipe, and cigar) between puffs and is not directly inhaled by the smoker; the smoke that gives rise to passive inhalation on the part of bystanders.

Sister chromatid exchange (SCE) Reciprocal exchange of chromatin between two replicated chromosomes that remain attached to each other until anaphase of mitosis; used as a measure of mutagenicity of substances that produce this effect.

Skeletal fluorosis Osteosclerosis due to fluoride.

Structure–activity relationship (SAR) Association between the physico-chemical properties of a substance and/or the properties of its molecular substructures and its biological properties including its toxicity.

Subacute (sometimes called subchronic) effect Biological change resulting from multiple or continuous exposures usually occurring over about 21 days. Sometimes the term is used synonymously with subchronic effect and care should be taken to check the usage any particular case.

Subchronic Related to repeated dose exposure over a short period, usually about 10% of the life span; an imprecise term used to describe exposures of intermediate duration.

Subchronic toxicity

1 Adverse effects resulting from repeated dosage or exposure to a substance over a short period, usually about 10% of the life span.

2 The capacity to produce adverse effects following subchronic exposure.

Subchronic (sometimes called subacute) toxicity test Animal experiment serving to study the effects produced by the test material when administered in repeated doses (or continually in food, drinking-water, air) over a period of about 90 days.

Surrogate Relatively well studied toxicant whose properties are assumed to apply to an entire chemically and toxicologically related class; for example, benzo(a)pyrene data may be used as toxicologically equivalent to that for all carcinogenic polynuclear aromatic hydrocarbons.

Symptom   Any subjective evidence of a disease or an effect induced by a substance as perceived by the affected subject.

Symptomatology   General description of all of the signs and symptoms of exposure to a toxicant; signs are the overt (observable) responses associated with exposure (such as convulsions, death, etc.) whereas symptoms are covert (subjective) responses (such as nausea, headache, etc.).

Syndrome   Set of signs and symptoms occurring together and often characterising a particular disease-like state.

Synergism   Pharmacological or toxicological interaction in which the combined biological effect of two or more substances is greater than expected on the basis of the simple summation of the toxicity of each of the individual substances.

Systemic   Relating to the body as a whole.

Systemic effect   Consequence that is of either a generalised nature or that occurs at the site distant from the point of entry of a substance: a systemic effect requires absorption and distribution of the substance in the body.

Target (of environmental pollution)   Human being or any organism, organ tissue cell, resource, or any constituent of the environment, living or not, that is subject to the activity of a pollutant or other chemical or physical activity or other agent.

Target organ(s)   Organ(s) in which the toxic injury manifests itself in terms of dysfunction or overt disease.

Teratogen   Agent that, when administered prenatally (to the mother), induces permanent structural malformations or defects in the offspring.

Teratogenicity   Potential to cause or the production of structural malformations or defects in offspring.

Testing of chemical
   1   In toxicology, evaluation of the therapeutic and potentially toxic effects of substances by their

application through relevant routes of exposure with appropriate organisms or biological systems so as to related effects to dose following application.

2   In chemistry, qualitative or quantitative analysis by the application of one or more fixed methods and comparison of the results with established standards.

Threshold Dose or exposure concentration below which an effect is not expected.

Threshold limit value (TLV) Concentration in air of a substance to which it is believed that most workers can be exposed daily without adverse effect (the threshold between safe and dangerous concentrations). These values are established (and revised annually) by the American Conference of Governmental Industrial Hygienists and are time-weighted concentrations for a 7 or 8 hour workday and a 40 hour workweek. For most substances the value may be exceeded, to a certain extent, provided there are compensatory periods of exposure below the value during the workday (or in some case the week). For a few substances (mainly those that produce a rapid response) the limit is given as a ceiling concentration (maximum permissible concentration – designated by "C") that should never be exceeded.

Tidal volume Quantity of air or test gas that is inhaled and exhaled during one respiratory cycle.

Time-weighted average exposure (TWAE) or concentration (TWAC) Concentration in the exposure medium at each measured time interval multiplied by time interval and divided by the total time of observation: for occupational exposure, working shift of eight hours is commonly used as the averaging time.

Tinnitus Continual noise in the ears, such as ringing, buzzing, roaring, or clicking.

Tissue dose Amount of a substance or physical agent (radiation) absorbed by a tissue.

Tolerable daily intake (TDI) Regulatory value equivalent to the acceptable daily intake established by the European Commission Scientific Committee on Food. Unlike the ADI, the TDI is expressed in mg/person, assuming a body weight of 60 kg. TDI normally used for food contaminants.

Tolerable risk Probability of suffering disease or injury that can, for the time being be tolerated, taking into account the associated benefits, and assuming that the risk is minimised by appropriate control procedures.

Tolerance

1   Adaptive state characterised by diminished effects of a particular dose of a substance: the process leading to tolerance is called "adaptation".

2   In food toxicology, dose that an individual can tolerate without showing an effect.

3   Ability to experience exposure to potentially harmful amounts of a substance without showing an adverse effect.

4   Ability of an organism to survive in the presence of a toxic substance: increased tolerance may be acquired by adaptation to constant exposure.

5   In immunology, state of specific immunological unresponsiveness.

Total diet study

1   Study designed to establish the pattern of pesticide residue intake by a person consuming a defined diet.

2   Study undertaken to show the range and amount of various foodstuffs in the typical diet or to estimate the total amount of a specific substance in a typical diet.

Toxicodynamics Process of interaction of potentially toxic substances with target and the biochemical and physiological consequences leading to adverse effects.

Toxicogenetics Study of the influence of hereditary factors on the effects of potent toxic substances on individual organisms.

Toxicokinetics Process of the uptake of potentially toxic substances by the body. The biotransformation in which they undergo the distribution of the substances and their metabolism. The tissues, and the elimination of the substances and their metabolites from the body. Both the amounts and the concentrations of the substances and their metabolites are studied. The term has essentially the same meaning as pharmaco-kinetics, but the latter term should be restricted to the study of pharmaceutical substances.

Toxicology   Scientific discipline involving the study of the actual or potential danger presented by the harmful effects of substances (poisons) on living organisms and ecosystems, of the relationship of such harmful effects to exposure, and of the mechanisms of action, diagnosis, prevention and treatment of intoxications.

Tracer

1   Means by which something may be followed; for example a radioactive isotope may replace a stable chemical element in a toxic compound enabling the toxicokinetics to be followed.

2   Labelled member of a population used to measure certain properties of that population.

Transformation

1   Alteration of a cell by incorporation of foreign genetic material and its subsequent expression in a new phenotype.

2   Conversion of cells growing normally to a state of rapid division in culture resembling that of a tumour.

3   Chemical modification of substances in the environment.

Transgenic   Adjective used to describe animals carrying a gene introduced by micro-injecting DNA into the nucleus of the fertilised egg.

Triage   Assessment of sick, wounded and injured persons following a disaster to determine priority needs for efficient use of available medical facilities.

Trophic level   Amount of energy in terms of food that an organism needs: organisms not needing organic food, such as plants, are said to be on a low trophic level, whereas predator species needing food of high energy content are said to be on a high trophic level. The trophic level indicates the level of the organism in the food chain.

Tumour
1   Any abnormal swelling or growth of tissue, whether benign or malignant.
2   Any abnormal growth, in rate and structure, that arises from normal tissue, but serves no physiological function.

Tumour progression   Sequence of changes by which a benign tumour develops the initial lesion to a malignant stage.

Ulcer   Defect, often associated with inflammation, occurring locally or at the surface, an organ or tissue owing to sloughing of necrotic tissue.

Validity (of a measurement)   Expression of the degree to which a measurement measures what it purports to measure.

Vasoconstriction   Decrease of the calibre of the blood vessels leading to a decreased blood flow.

Vasodilation   Increase in the calibre of the blood vessels, leading to an increased blood flow.

Ventilation
1   Process of supplying a building or room with fresh air.
2   Process of exchange of air between the ambient atmosphere and the lungs.
3   In physiology, the amount of air inhaled per day.
4   Oxygenation of blood.

Ventricular fibrillation   Irregular heartbeat characterised by uncoordinated contractions of the ventricle.

Volume of distribution   Apparent (hypothetical) volume of fluid required to contain the total amount of a substance in the body at the same concentration as that present in the plasma assuming equilibrium has been attained.

Weight-of-evidence for toxicity Extent to which the available biomedical data support the hypothesis that a substance causes a defined toxic effect such as cancer in humans.

Further reading on pathology

Abbas, A. K., Lichtman, A. H. and Pober, J. S. (2000) *Cellular and molecular immunology*, 4th edn, Orlando: W. B. Saunders Company.

Alison, M. R. and Sarraf, C. E. (eds) (1997) *Understanding cancer*, Cambridge: Cambridge University Press.

Alison, M. R. and Sarraf, C. E. (1995) "Apoptosis: regulation and relevance to toxicology", *Human and Experimental Toxicology* 14: 234–247.

Alberts, B., Bray, D., Lewis, J., Raff, M., Roberts, K. and Watson, J. (1983) *The molecular biology of the cell*, New York: Garland Publishing.

Anderson, D. and Conning, D. (eds) (1993) *Experimental toxicology, the basic issues*, 2nd edn, London: Royal Society of Chemistry.

Anderson, J. H. (ed.) (1980) *Muir's textbook of pathology*, London: Edward Arnold.

Benjamini, E., Coico, R. and Sunshine, G. (2000) *Immunology: a short course*, 4th edn, London: Wiley & Sons Inc.

Clark, B. and Smith, D. (eds) (1993) *An introduction to pharmacokinetics*, London Blackwell Scientific Publications.

Corcoran, G. B., Fix, L., Jones, D. B., Moslen, M. T., Nicotera, P., Oberhamer, F. A. and Buttaya, R. (1994) "Molecular control point in Toxicology", *Toxicology and Applied Pharmacology* 128: 169–181.

Glaister, J. R. (ed.) (1986) *Principals of toxicological pathology*, London: Taylor and Francis.

Goldsby, R. A., Kindt, T. J. and Osborne, B. A. (2000) *Kuby immunology*, 4th edn, London: W. H. Freeman & Company.

Govan, D. T., McFarlane, P. S. and Callander, R. (1995) *Pathology illustrated*, London and New York: Churchill & Livingstone.

Grasso, P., Sharratt M. and Cohen, A. J. (1991) "Role of persistent non-genotoxic tissue damage in rodent cancer and its relevance", in: *Annual review of pharmacology and toxicology* vol. 31, California, USA.

Grasso, P. (1992) "Testing for carcinogenicity", in: *Experimental toxicology – the basic issues*, 2nd Edn, The Royal Society of Chemistry, London.

Hoffbrand, A. V. and Pettit, J. E. (2001) *Essential haematology*, 4th edn, Oxford: Blackwell Science.

Howard, M. R. and Hamilton, P. J. (1997) *Haematology – an illustrated colour text*, London: Churchill Livingstone.

Kumar, V., Cotran, R. and Robbins, S. (eds) (1997) *Basic pathology*, London, NewYork: W. P. Saunders.

Lakhani, S. R., Dilly, S. A. and Finlayson, C. J. (1998) *Basic pathology: an introduction to the mechanisms of disease*, 2nd edn, London: Arnold Publishers.

Levin, S. (1998) "Apoptosis, Necrosis, Oncosis: What is your diagnosis?" A report from the cell death nomenclature committee of the Society of Toxicological Pathologists Science 41: 115–116.

Lodish, H., Berk, A., Zipursky, L., Matsudaira, P., Baltimore D. and Darnell, J. (2000) *Molecular cell biology*, 4th edn, New York: W. H. Freeman & Company.

Mathews, C. K., van Holde, K. E. and Ahern, K. G. (1999) *Biochemistry*, 3rd edn, San Francisco: Addison Wesley.

Pallister, C. (1994) *Blood physiology and pathophysiology*, London: Arnold Publishers.

Spector, W. G. and Spector, T. (eds) (1989) *An introduction to general pathology*, London and New York: Churchill Livingstone.

Stevens, A. and Lowe, J. (1995) *Pathology*, 2nd edn, London: Mosby.

Stevens, A. and Lowe, J. (2000) *Pathology illustrated review in color*, 2nd edn, London: Mosby.

Stryer, L. (1995) *Biochemistry*, 4th edn, New York: W. H. Freeman & Company.

Timbrell, J. A. (ed.) (1997) *Introduction to toxicology*, London: Taylor & Francis.

Turton, J. and Hooson, J. (eds) (1998) *Target organ pathology: a basic text*, London: Taylor & Francis.

Underwood, J. C. E. (2000) *General and systematic pathology*, 3rd edn, London: Churchill Livingstone.

Voet, D. and Voet, J. G. (1995) *Biochemistry*, 2nd edn, New York: John Wiley & Sons Inc.

Walters, J. B. and Isreal, M. P. (1969) *General pathology*, London and New York: J & A Churchill.

Willis, R. (1967) *Pathology of tumours*, 4th edn, London Melbourne and New York: Blackwell.

Yarnold, J. R., Stratton, M. and McMillan T. J. (eds) (1996) *Molecular biology for oncologists*, 2nd edn, London: Chapman and Hall.

Further reading on clinical chemistry

Develin, T. M. (ed.) (1997) *Textbook of biochemistry – with clinical correlations*, 4th edn, London: Wiley – Liss Inc.

Gray, C. J., Howorth, P. J. and Rinsier, M. J. (1996) *Clinical chemical pathology*, 10th edn, London: Edward Arnold.

Smith, A. F., Beckett, G. J., Walker, S. W. and Roe, P. W. H. (1998) *Lecture notes on clinical biochemistry*, Oxford: Blackwell Science.

Holme, D. J. and Peck, H. (1993) *Analytical biochemistry*, 2nd edn, Harlow: Longman Scientific and Technical, Longman Group UK Ltd.

Hooson, J. and Turton, J. (eds) (1998) *Target organ pathology: a basic text*, London: Taylor and Francis.

Laker, M. F. (1996) *Clinical biochemistry for medical students*, London: W. B. Saunders Co Ltd.

Bloomfield, M. B. (1992) *Chemistry and the living organism*, 5th edn, New York: John Wiley and Sons Inc.

Varley, H., Gowenlock, A. H. and Bell, M. (1980) *Practical clinical biochemistry*, 5th edn, 2 vols., London: William Heinemann Medical Books Ltd.

Toniolo, P., Boffetta, P., Shuker, D. E. G., Rothman, N., Hulka, B. and Pearce, N. (eds) (1997) *"Application of biomarkers in cancer epidemiology"*. IARC scientific publication No. 142, International Agency for Research on Cancer, Lyon.

IEH report on the use of biomarkers in environmental exposure assessment Report R5 (1996) Institute for environment and health, Medical Research Council, Leicester.

Gangolli, S. and Phillips, J. C. (1993) "The metabolism and disposition of xenobiotics", in: D. Anderson and D. M. Conning (eds) *Experimental toxicology – The basic issues*, 2nd edn, Royal Society of Chemistry, Cambridge.

Klaasen, C. D. (ed.) (1996) "The basic science of poisons", in: *Casarett and Doull's toxicology*, New York: McGraw – Hill Companies Inc.

Ballantyne, B., Marrs, T. C. and Syversen, T. (1999) *General and applied toxicology*, 2nd edn, 3 vols., Basingstoke: Macmillan References Ltd.

Further reading on haematology

Brantom, P. G., Gaunt, I. F., Grasso, P., Lansdown, A. B. G and Gangolli, S. D. (1972) "Short-term toxicity of tolualdehyde in rats". *Food and Cosmetics Toxicology* 10: 637–647.

Gaunt, I. F. (1973) Studies on the Relationship Between Heinz Bodies and Haemolysis in Laboratory Animals and the Evaluation of Heinz Body Production in Toxicological Investigation. Ph.D. Thesis, University of London.

Gaunt, I. F. and Lane-Petter, W. (1967) "Vitamin K deficiency in 'SPF' rats". *Laboratory Animals* 1: 147–149.

Gaunt, I. F., Colley, J., Wright, M., Creasey, M., Grasso, P. and Gangolli, S. D. (1971) "Acute and short-term toxicity studies on *trans*-2-hexenal". *Food and Cosmetics Toxicology* 9: 775–786.

Gaunt, I. F., Hardy, J., Grasso, P., Gangolli, S. D. and Butterworth, K. R. (1976) "Long-term toxicity of cyclohexylamine hydrochloride in the rat". *Food and Cosmetics Toxicology* 14: 255–267.

Gaunt, I. F., Lloyd, A. G., Grasso, P. Gangolli, S. D. and Butterworth, K. R. (1977) "Short-term study in the rat on two caramels produced by variaions of the 'ammonia process'". *Food and Cosmetics Toxicology* 15: 509–521.

Marrs, T. C., Bright, J. E. and Morris, B. C. (1987) "Methemoglobinogenic potential of primaquine and its mutagenicity in the Ames test". *Toxicology Letters* 36: 281–287.

Winstanley, P. A., Mberu, E. K., Szwandt, I. S. F., Breckenridge, A. M. and Watkins, W. M. (1995) "*In vitro* activities of novel antifolate drug combinations against *Plasmodium falciparum* and human granulocyte CFUs". *Antimicrobial Agents Chemotherapy* 39: 948–952.

Index

acquired immunodeficiency
syndrome (AIDS) 43
adenocarcinoma 35
adenosine triphosphate (ATP) 59,
111, 138
adrenal 63, 72, 74, 75, 76, 78, 79,
80, 84
adrenocorticotropic hormone
(ACTH) 73, 74, 75, 79
alanine aminotransferase (ALT) 62,
76, 80
alkaline phosphatase (ALP) 62, 76,
80
allergy 43
alphafetoprotein (AFP) 72, 84
anaerobic glycolysis 59
angiotensin II (AII) 73, 75
annular tumour 35
antiprotease inhibitor (API) 70
arginine vasopressin (AVP) 73,
75
aspartate aminotransferase (AST)
62, 76, 80
autoimmunity 43

bile; acids 76; duct 11; pigments 9
bioactivation and detoxification
56, 63, 64, 66, 76, 83
biochemical changes related to
chemical toxicity 74–79;
hypothalamus-pituitary-adrenal
axis 78–79; methodology-
general 79–2

blood 17, 18, 20, 21, 22, 25, 32, 33,
37, 40, 50, 55, 59, 62, 68, 70, 71,
72, 74, 78, 81, 82, 84, 87–93,
95–98, 101, 104, 107, 110, 111,
113, 117, 122, 128, 130, 133,
134, 153; clot 17, 18, 26,
70, 71, 89, 91, 92, 96, 105, 128;
thrombus 17
butylated hydroxytoluene (BHT)
52

calcification; dystrophic 11;
metastatic 11
cancer 31–8; causation of
tumour 37; tissue growth
and 38; neoplasia 31;
histological characteristics 34–5;
taxonomy 32–4, 35–7;
mechanism of tumour
production 37–8
carcinoembryonic antigen (CEA)
72
carcinogenesis 54, 117, 127
catarrh 21
catecholamine 71, 74
cell and cell damage, The 1–9
cell damage short of death 4;
cytoplasm and its organelles
6–9; division 2–4; nucleus 4–6
cell damage, changes indicative
of 11–12; hyalyne 11; amyloid 12;
fibrinoid change 11–12
cell, age of 89, 98

cells, reactive responses of 14–16;
    atrophy 15; hyperplasia 15;
    hypertrophy 14; metaplasia 15;
    oedema 15–16
cellular pathology 1–16
central nervous system (CNS) 72,
    84
choriocarcinoma 72
chromosomal; rearrangement 54;
    translocation 54
chromosomes 4, 34, 45;
    aneuploidy 35
Clara cells 63
cloudy swelling 6, 8, 52
corticotropin releasing hormone
    (CRH) 73, 75
corticotropin-like intermediary
    peptide (CLIP) 74
creatine kinase (CK) 62, 67, 77, 80
cyanosis (blueness) 20
cytology 88–9

dehydroepiandrosterone
    (DHEA) 75
deoxyribonucleic acid (DNA) 1, 4,
    6, 53, 54, 59, 60, 81, 113, 114,
    118, 127, 130, 138, 140, 142, 145,
    152
desmoenzyme (cellular
    membrane) 57
dietary factors 47
dimethyl nitrosamine (DMN) 53
disease, causation 45–7; acquired-
    infective agents 46–7;
    congenital disease 47;
    genetically determined 45

electron microscope (EM) 6
embolism 18
endoplasmic reticulum (ER) 1, 8,
    60, 63, 122, 133, 139, 141;
    rough 1, 61; smooth 1, 61
enzyme-linked immunosorbent
    assay (ELISA) 81
enzymes 56–68; classification
    57–8; intracellular location
    59–63; nature and function
    56–57; structural variants and

cytochrome P-450 haemoprotein
    polymorphism 67–68; xenobiotic
    metabolism, involved 63–7
enzyme–substrate 57, 67
epithelial tumour; papilloma 35
ethylenediamine tetra-acetic acid
    (EDTA) 91
extracellular fluid (ECF) 15;
    exudate 16; transudate 16;
exudative 21

fat 1, 8, 9, 10, 82, 110
fibrosarcoma/fibroma 35, 37
fibrosis 21; cystic 78
fibrous histiocytoma, malignant 37
follicle-stimulating hormone (FSH)
    73, 74, 75

gamma-glutamyl transferase
    (GGT) 62, 76, 80
gangrene; dry 14, 18; wet 12, 18
gene amplification 54
genotoxic 6, 96
Giemsa method 95
glucose-6-phosphate
    dehydrogenase (G-6-PD) 98
gonadotropin release inhibiting
    factor (GnRIF) 73
gonadotropin releasing hormone
    (GnRH) 73, 75
growth hormone (GH) 73, 75

haemangiosarcoma/haemangioma
    37
haematology and toxicology
    studies 89–98; factors affecting
    quality 91–3; historical data 93–8
haemophilia 45
haemorrhagic 21
haemosiderin 9
heart 9, 17, 50, 51, 52, 62, 67, 77,
    80, 111
Heinz bodies 97, 98
Hodgkin's disease 12
human chorionic gonadotropin
    (hCG) 72
human immunodeficiency virus
    (HIV) 43

5-hydroxyindole acetic acid
(5-HIAA) 71
hyperaemia 20
hyperchromasia 35

immunoglobin G (IgG) 72
immunoglobulin 70, 71, 72, 77, 83
immunology 39–44; acquired
(specific) immunity 41;
B-lymphocytes 41–2; innate
(non-specific) immunity 39–41;
T-lymphocytes 42–3;
infarction 17, 18
inflammation; acute 18–21;
chronic 21–5
international union of
biochemistry and molecular
biology (IUBMB) 57
interstitial fluid (IF) 20
isoenzymes 67

kidney 8, 46, 62, 63, 70, 77, 78, 79,
80, 84, 114, 124, 140
Kwashiorkor 47

lactate dehydrogenase (LDH) 16,
62, 67, 77, 80
lactogenic hormone (LH) 73
leiomyosarcoma/leiomyoma 37
lipofuscin 9
β-lipotropin (β-LTH) 74
liver 8, 9, 11, 46, 51, 52, 61, 62, 63,
67, 68, 70, 71, 76, 80, 83, 97, 113,
133
Lupus vulgaris 37
luteinizing hormone (LH) 74, 75
lysoenzymes (Free soluble
enzymes) 57
lysosomes 1, 2, 3, 52, 59, 60, 107,
134, 141

major histo-compatibility complex
(MHC) 42
Marjolin's ulcer 37
meiosis 4, 45
melanin 9
methhaemoglobin 98
β₂-microglobulin 70, 71

mitochondria 1, 2, 4, 8, 52, 59, 60,
61, 138
mitosis 4
mixed function oxidase (MFO) 56,
61, 69, 138

necrobiosis 51
necrosis and apoptosis 12–14
nephrotic syndrome 84
NAD(P)H (nicotinamideadenine-
dinucleotide (phosphate)H) 60, 61

pancreas 62, 74, 75, 76, 78
pathology 49–54; adaptation 52–3;
apoptosis 51–2; oncogenes
53–4; other genetic activity 54;
recurrent themes 50–1; target
organ toxicity 53
peroxisomes 1, 2, 52, 59, 60, 61, 141
phagocytes 40, 41
physiologically-based
pharmacokinetic (PBPK) 67
pituitary 38, 72, 75, 76, 78, 80, 84;
anterior 73, 79, 84; posterior 79
plasma; hormones and steroids
in 72–4; proteins in 68–72
platelets 17, 87, 89, 91, 94, 95, 96
point mutation 54
polyp 35
prions (protein) 46
programmed cell death (PCD) 51
progressive tissue damage 9–11
prolactin (PRL) 38, 73, 74, 75, 79
prolactin release inhibiting factor
(PIF) 73
prolactin releasing factor (PRF) 73,
75
prostate specific antigen (PSA) 72,
84
pulmonary tuberculosis 9
pyknosis (nucleus) 8

RNA (ribonucleic acid) 59, 60, 61,
127, 130, 145
rubella virus (German measles) 47

sarcoma 35
somatocrinin (GRH) 73, 75

somatostatin (GIH) 73, 75
squamous cell carcinoma 35
storage disorders 11
suppurative 21

T-cell receptor (TCR) 42
T-cytotoxic (T$_C$) 41
T-helper (T$_H$) 41
thrombosis 17–18
thyroid gland 72, 75, 76, 78, 80, 84
thyrotropin or thyroid stimulating hormone (TSH) 73, 75, 80
thyrotropin releasing hormone (TRH) 73, 75
thyroxine (T$_4$) 70, 71, 74, 75, 78, 80

tissue injury 25–9; repair 27–9; restitution 25–7
tissue-specific toxicity 87
transitional cell carcinoma 35
tri-iodothyronine (T$_3$) 71, 74, 75, 78, 80
Tumour; biological behaviour 31; enchephaloid 35; macroscopic appearance 32; scirrhous 35

ultraviolet light type B (UVB) 45

varicose ulcers 37

Wilson's disease 70, 84

Xeroderma pigmentosum 45